The Strength of a Man
The Journey of a Cancer Warrior

DERRICK CAMERON

To request permission, contact the publisher at kingdpublishing@gmail.com

ISBN: 978-1-7356459-0-2

First edition October 2020.

Edit and layout by Shonell Bacon

Book cover designed by Barbara Upshaw-Mayers

Cover art by Dokk Savage Photography and Richie Carter Photography

Printed in the United States of America.

DEDICATION

To everyone associated in the fight for life,

I wrote about my experiences so that it may inspire everyone who reads my story to push forward regardless of the perceived health status. Anyone going through cancer most likely will encounter some level of depression and will need encouragement. Caregivers need support just as much as the cancer warriors. A lot of times, caregivers struggle with the loving desire to help but lack the full understanding of the experience. This is challenging in multiple levels. This book will hopefully give some insight to those who serve in the caregivers position. This is also for the friends and support groups who may not fully understand as well. I hope that the words expressed in this book will serve as guidance for supporting those who may have to go through, or is going through, or have gone through the battle of cancer.

CONTENTS

ACKNOWLEDGMENTS

I must start by thanking my awesome mother who was there every step of the journey. She was so loving, caring, patient, willing to learn, and driven to help me stay on track with my medical requirements. I love you. I am extending a special thank you to Jeramiah Jackson for being an inspiration. You have always shown me love for being me in good and in bad. Thank you to my UAH colleagues who consistently visited, texted, and called: Shaun Perry, Kim Battle, Aisha Chambliss, Brent Bell and family, Laffon Brelland, Robert Sawyer, Vence Lett, and Ryan Wilson.

To my closer friends from life experiences, I thank you for your expressions of love as well. Thank you to Laura Love for being my inspiration to push forward through the rough times. Thank you to Shameka McCoy, Lavon White, Terrance Pitts, Rod Hill, Tasha & Xavier Hereford, Anthony & Debra Coleman, Al Stanley, and Anthony Lancaster. Thank you to all my friends and colleagues whom I did not specifically list. I appreciate each action of love that you extended.

Thank you to Hundley Batts Sr. for your motivation to reach out and be a voice for those who choose not or cannot speak out about cancer. In memory of the late Russell Brown, owner of DP Associates, thank you for your guidance to my professional career by sharing your life experiences. Thank you to Jerrod Young who provided me with life experiences that have helped me develop mental fortitude. Thank you to my dad for your expressions of love. Claudinette Purifoy-Fears, you have helped me chase dreams and held me accountable for the responsibility to keep reaching back. In memory of the late Dr. Adriel Johnson—he was a great educator of life and definitely had a personality that would challenge your critical thinking. I loved him for that.

I want to also thank Clearview Cancer Institute for the great care and love shown to me during my chemotherapy treatments. Thanks to the Sierra Lobo Inc. team members who donated their Personal Time Off hours to me so I may take off work as needed during my chemotherapy treatments. Thank you to Dr. James K. Olszewski and the Rocket City Chiropractic staff. Dr. O helped me get my spine aligned so my spinal cord would be in the best possible state to support my immune system. Thank you to the National Society of Black Engineers Alumni–North Alabama Chapter for supporting me during my time as president. Everyone stepped up so we could still positively impact the community without missing a beat. Thank you to the Ruff Ryders (RR)–Huntsville chapter who treated me like an honorary brother. In the RR specifically, Steve "ATL" Pearson, Willie "Old School" Applewhite, "Brooklyn," "Snapper," and the late "750's" mother.

Thank you to everyone who helped me get this book to print. I want to thank Marc Lacy for guiding me through the process. Thank you, Shonell Bacon, for editing the book. Thank you to Barbara Upshaw-Mayers for putting together a great book cover. Thank you to Dokk Savage Photography and Richie Carter for working with me to get the necessary pictures.

A MESSAGE FROM MOTHER

Who is a true survivor? Derrick.

One day, he woke up, and his world had changed forever. He was faced with a reality he never dreamed possible. It was his worst nightmare, and his world was crumbling around him. Determined not to be a victim to anyone or anything, he decided to set a new course for his life. He redesigned himself, his life, and his environment to create a life for the future. It won't be easy. It will be an uphill climb from the start. But the view he now has is worth every struggle he faced. He will become the man he always wanted to be. Strong, yet tender. Wise, yet humble. Open, loving, and forgiving, not letting any of the past hold him down. He never dreamed the devastation he once faced would be the refiner's fire that turned his life around. Derrick is now the epitome of a true survivor. I love you.

Hattie Gibby Cameron

CHAPTER 1 | PERSONAL FOUNDATION

I was the product of a drill sergeant dad in the United States Army and a southern God-fearing mother. My dad is from North Carolina, and my mother is from Alabama. A little boy born in New Jersey, I was destined to have an anointed and interesting life. It turns out that my mother was pregnant for six months without knowing she was pregnant. She had every indication that she was not pregnant until she went to the doctor because she was gaining weight. She then started preparing for my arrival. I would be the first surviving child in three pregnancies.

My father was serving the United States Army when I was born. His career was the catalyst for a multitude of events that helped shaped my personality. As a kid, we traveled a lot over half of the world. We also moved a lot, so it became normal that we did not try to get too close to friends that we made. We knew we would be picking everything up to move within a year or two. All of the traveling made me very capable of adapting to multiple cultures and adjusting to various environments. These are traits that actually helped advance and sustain my career as I got older. Traveling has always created great memories throughout my youth. I could remember so many things even at a very young age.

I have always had a good memory. I remember our family being in New Jersey when I was a baby and laying in my crib looking up at my mother and father standing over me. I remember so much of my childhood. We were always traveling to different states. My mother had nine siblings and my dad had three siblings. My dad's siblings were all in North Carolina; however, my mother's siblings left the country of southern Alabama over time.

During our first stint in Baumholder, Germany, one of my mother's older brother and her first cousin were both stationed in Germany at the same time. I was about five years old. My mother's cousin Brenda was one of my favorite family members. She was a body builder and Golden Gloves boxer in the army. She used to teach me how to box when I was little. She bought me a pair of boxing gloves and would occasionally take me to one of the gyms she trained at in Germany.

While in Germany, I had other great experiences like walking to elementary school across what seemed like a huge field in the snow. The kids at the German schools were real fun. Although I was a minority in the schools in Germany, my classmates were always nice to me throughout the years we were overseas. I remember that there was a Santa riding a reindeer-pulled sleigh through the neighborhood. I played little league football, basketball, and soccer not far from the neighborhood. I remember traveling the countryside often by bus, train, and car. One time, we had an accident on the Autobahn, resulting in Mother having to go to a German hospital. German hospitals did not resemble what you would expect in the States. It was just like something you would see in an old war movie.

My dad had a Porsche, and we would go riding on the Autobahn all the time. One time, we went joy riding and went to an area that the solders would go to hang out. It was wet one particular day, and we got stuck somewhat off the road. We spent hours trying to get that Porsche 911 out of the mud.

We eventually moved back to the States when I was about seven years old, where I continued to play little league sports. I picked up coach-pitch baseball and swimming to go along with my other three sports. I definitely was active everywhere that we stayed.

Every U.S. location we were stationed in brought new expected and unexpected challenges. I knew I would have to make new friends, but I was unaware that there was going to be some unexpected treatment coming from kids my age. When we returned to the States, we were stationed in Oak Ridge, NC. In that time, I witnessed and experienced more than my share of racism. The school I attended did not even have another minority there. The only time I saw minorities my age was when we played other towns in little league basketball, football, or baseball. There were times that a lot of the boys would try to gang up to try and extort me for items or bully me. I always would keep quiet and try to walk away except for the one time when about five of them followed me to the bathroom and tried to jump me.

I turned around, and the door was blocked. My heart started racing because I could see the evil in their young eyes. When the first boy walked up and tried to hit me, I ducked and followed up with two punches. When he fell, I hit each of the other two immediately behind him. With an opening created, I ran and returned to the playground. I just knew I was going to get called to the office, but I never did, and after that, I never had a problem from those boys again. However, each year, another set of boys would see how far they could push me. It was funny that these boys never played sports because the boys that I played sports with never gave me any problems to the extent that I dared call them my friends.

I really believe I got my baseball skills from my mother's father. He was a skillful pitcher, but he never had a strikeout as a batter that any of his children can remember. He loved fast-pitch baseball. I like to think a little of his baseball skills were passed down through my bloodline. My mother was a track star in her community. I definitely had a lot of athletic family members on that side of my family. My grandfather was the pillar of the family and one of a few for the community. He was a God-fearing man who really cherished his family. He taught his grandchildren the same things he taught his children, which were to be respectable, family oriented, and responsible. In a way, he was the first to teach me teamwork because he taught us that the family should always stick together through thick and thin. He would give me history lessons about the family and share his wisdom with me all the time. I really would pattern my life around his teachings. The beginning of my efforts to mimic my mother's father was by playing sports wherever I was located.

My sports activity level started dropping off as I got older. In middle school, I played football for the school but played city league basketball and baseball. I stopped playing soccer and swimming. When I got to high school, I played football and basketball for the school my first two years. I had stopped playing baseball, however, by the time I got to high school.

Eventually, I stopped playing sports so I would have the opportunity to get a job and help my mother pay the household bills.

I remember having to tell my high school football coach that I was going to have to quit playing football to get a job. As I told him why I was getting the job, he asked me was I sure what I was doing. I told him I felt like this was what I had to do. I will never forget the look on his face. Although he was always carrying a mean look on his face, and none of the over filled testosterone guys would test Coach McGuire, a look of concern filled him. This was the one moment that it seemed like the guy who I felt was heartless for making me do the 200 grass drills for allegedly disrupting a class, became human. I never got in trouble in school because I was more scared of my mother's response than I was of anyone else, so I welcomed the football punishment. I also welcomed the subtle emotional response from the coach who I know had a bunch of unasked questions.

It was very emotional having to quit playing the sports that I so loved. However, since I was in a single-parent home, it was harder watching my mother struggle to keep food on the table. I already had a little part time job, cleaning an office twice a week (Wednesday and Saturday) since I was 12. I got the job to start saving for my first car. That cleaning job paid me approximately $75 weekly. When I was 16, I made the decision to bring in some money to help stabilize the home. I picked up another job at Kenny Rogers Roasters. I worked there until they shut the doors a year later, and then I picked up another job at a parts store. The summer after my senior year, I picked up another part-time job at a local community center where I met some great people. It turned out to be wonderful opportunities that led to another summer job with a Builders' Association.

Working with the Builders' Association allowed me to meet a lot of local business owners and to get a better understanding of how to be an entrepreneur. While working there, I learned of other opportunities to assist my college endeavors. I originally wanted to be an architect because I loved to draw. I wanted to go to a Historically Black College or University. After looking at the scholarships that I had won and was offered at the schools and the cost of getting the degree, it was more economical for me to follow my second choice of being an electrical engineer. So, after winning a reoccurring scholarship from the Builders' Association, I asked them to push the scholarship to the University of Alabama in Huntsville where I would obtain my bachelor's degree in electrical engineering. After graduation, I immediately followed it up with my master's in management of technology.

To this day, I have cherished the relationships that I have established with all the professionals that I have made along the way. I have met people who work in the automotive world racing, fixing, and building cars. I love customizing and detailing my own vehicles. Customizing can be frustrating, and sometimes you will get injured, but the final product is something you can be proud of. Relationships with other car enthusiasts were born along the way. I established just as many relationships with people I met at the gym and while playing intramural sports. I continued to play intramural and city league sports after I graduated because I love competition between others and against myself. My competitive spirit drives me through many situations.

CHAPTER 2 | WHAT IS THAT?

Playing flag football was a normal activity I participated in annually during and after college. It was the only intramural sport that I had not won a championship in up to 2009. I have been on different teams that had made it to the championship game, but we could never cross that hump. I felt like I was on the Buffalo Bills team of the 1990s. Despite that, our 2009 Blackhawks team was special because it was so diverse. The team was made up of a lot of alumni and guys who trained in the school's fitness center. We were a strong group of guys that had great cohesion.

Flag football can be a physical contact sport. During the season that ran from August to November, I played on the offensive line against one of the more talented teams in the league. This particular team had a strong defensive line. There were some serious battles in the trenches while we tried to keep those strong defensive players from our quarterback. There were plenty of elbows and forearms to each other. It was not a surprise to go home feeling beat up. In the middle of the season, I would go home with several bruises.

When I got home after a game in October 2009, I walked through the door, put my gym bag down by my washer machine, and headed over to the island to get a large pot. As I put my left hand on the island and reached with my right hand inside the island, I felt what seemed like a muscle strain in the left side of my chest. I started rubbing the left side of my chest, thinking, *Dang, that hurts.* I didn't think much more about it at the time.

While the oven started to get warm, and the water in the pot started to boil, I decided to take a quick shower. In my normal routine, I went to my bedroom, turned on some music, started the shower, and began to pull off my clothes. As I pulled off my shirt, I looked in the mirror and saw a bruise. I came home with yet another one. This particular bruise was on my left pectoral muscle, and it was very noticeable against my caramel complexion. It was black and blue and about 3 inches in diameter, sitting just above the nipple. I really did not notice that the bruise was that deep until I looked in the mirror. I figured it would take about a week for that one to go away. I jumped in the shower and lathered up, not giving my bruises much consideration thereafter.

During the week, every time I would take a shower, I would continue to rub my chest and feel the spot where I got hit. I noticed what felt like a small knot under the skin. I figured it was just part of the injury, so I kept things moving.

By the next game, the color where the injury occurred had returned to that of my skin tone. The soreness from the injury started to go away. In the second week after noticing the bruise, I was in the shower and rubbed then massaged my left chest with my forefinger and middle finger together. I noticed what felt like a harden knot about the size of a pea. I was not sure what this thing was, but I started to think that it might just go away. The attitude I carried ever since I was in middle school was that if I could do anything instead of going to a doctor, then that was what I would do. I never did like going to the doctor. I tried to avoid them at all costs. So, in this situation, I didn't think this little knot warranted a visit to the doctor. As the weeks went on, I kept feeling this pea-sized knot under my skin. After about three to four weeks, I noticed that the knot did not go away, so I decided that I would go to the doctor after the season ended.

The final Sunday of the season, which was the second Sunday before Thanksgiving, we were playing in the Championship game. It was a hard-fought game between the two best teams in the league. When the last whistle blew, the Blackhawks were victorious, and I finally got a championship in the one intramural sport that eluded me while I was attending college. I was feeling real good that we were able to pull out the tough win. I remember taking a team picture after we got our T-shirts, shaking hands with all the guys on the team, and saying that we would do it again next year. I got in my car, feeling good, and turned up the music for my journey home.

When I got home and put my stuff down by the washer, I proceeded to my bedroom so I could take a shower. After I got in the shower, I felt the same area that I had been monitoring. I rubbed my chest with close attention and thought the knot felt bigger. Now, I was a little more concerned. I looked down at my chest where the knot was, and I took my forefinger and thumb and pinched the area. Using my forefinger and my thumb, I tried to bring the two together under the knot so that it would push up the knot to the skin level so I could determine the real size of it. I could tell that there was an outline of something, but it was not clear what it was. I squeezed it a little bit, and it appeared to be solid. It definitely was not any sort of liquid substance. Next, I took my forefinger and pushed at the skin next to the area where the knot was and tried to push as if I wanted to push the knot from the bottom. The pea-sized knot seemed to move under the skin about a quarter of an inch, but then it would return back to the same area. I pushed on it from what seemed like every direction, and I could see the outline of this thing under my skin. I remember saying to myself, "I definitely need to contact the doctor tomorrow."

The following day while at work, I contacted my family doctor to set up an appointment for later in the week. After I received confirmation of the appointment, I thought, *I can't wait to get this over with.*

The day of the appointment arrived, and I left work to travel approximately 20 minutes to get to the doctor's office early. When I got there, at least 15 minutes early no mind, I checked in then waited to be called. There was a room full of people there, and all the patients looked like they were there to battle some type of cold. There were pharmaceutical representatives there as well. Now, with all these people in the building and only two doctors on duty, how were we going to keep the schedule? While we were sitting there, I heard a lady say that she was going to be late getting back to work. She said that she came early for her 10 o'clock appointment, and she still had not gone to the back. I then proceeded to ask her, "Who is your doctor?" Interesting enough, she had the same doctor I had, at the exact same appointment time. Now, looking at the number of people that were in there to see one of the two doctors and the number of rooms in the back, a thorough analysis of the patient throughput was not completed. A little after 11 o'clock, I finally went to the back to get all my vitals and wait in the little room by myself. I often used this time to take a nice nap before the doctor came in because I knew I would have plenty of time.

Eventually, the doctor came in and asked how I was doing. I told him I was fine and that I was here to get a knot on my chest checked out. He told me to take off my shirt so he could examine the area in my chest. After taking off my shirt, he began to push on my chest at the area I pointed out. He stated that he would like to do an ultrasound of the area to see if it truly was a mass.

"Men usually get tumors in various places in the body," he said, "but most of them are benign."

At this point, I was somewhat confident in what he was saying because of our relationship outside of the office. The doctor came to the fitness center at my alma mater at 6 o'clock in the weekday mornings to play basketball, so I had a greater level of trust in what he was saying because of our friendship.

He ordered an ultrasound for the latter part of the following week at the same facility. Before I departed, he reassured me that I most likely had nothing to worry about.

The following week, I went for the ultrasound at the doctor's office. When I got in the back, they asked me to pull my shirt off and lay down on the table. So, I pulled off my shirt, and lay down on the very cold table. The lights were already dimmed when I walked into the room. I remember thinking that I could go to sleep in there if he did not move swiftly. The technician told me that he had to put this gel on my chest that would be used for the ultrasound. He warned me that it could be rather cold at times. That statement was very true. The gel was cold, and I flexed my chest like I was at a body building contest when he applied it with his gloved hand.

In a humorous tone, he stated, "Looks like that the gel is cold."

"You think?" I responded.

After applying the gel, the technician wheeled over this fairly large machine on casters. He pulled from the machine what looked like a microphone-shaped wand with a coiled cord at the base and began to rub the sensor across my chest. As he began scanning my chest's surface, he adjusted the screen. While scanning the area of my chest where the mass was, he captured screenshots of the mass' location. After about 20 minutes of reapplying the cold gel and taking screenshots, the technician told me that I was done.

As I put my shirt back on, I asked him what was the next step.

He told me that he would send the pictures in for review, and afterwards, they will send the results to the doctor. The doctor would then contact me with the results.

The results came in at the beginning of the next week, and my doctor's office called me to come in to get my results. We made an appointment for the next day.

Again, I left work so that I could make it to doctor's office on time, and I still had to wait a substantial time for my appointment. I often wonder if they make you wait on purpose so that your blood pressure would be influenced to rise so they may put you on added medicine. Finally, I got my turn to wait in the little room. The doctor came in and went through the normal ritual of being cordial.

"The test results definitely appear to have evidence that a mass is present," he said.

"Ok, what is the next step?" I asked. I was not bothered, just confused. A mass could mean anything, but I thought it was a minimal thing to be concerned about at best.

"We need to have a biopsy completed. It's a way of sampling the mass. Since the mass is the size it is, it will not be difficult to remove."

He recommended a general surgeon, Dr. Fernandez, and stated that his office would set up the appointment for me. After asking me if I had any questions, I told him, "No, I don't have any questions."

He shook my hand—then, I didn't know that would be for the last time.

I proceeded to go to the checkout desk to get my appointment details. The lady behind the counter had a look of despair on her face because her coworker had gotten smart with her. She was an older lady that you knew did not have a high tolerance for the ignorance that was easily associated with a younger person who believed they knew everything. I was moved that she was on the edge of tears, so I decided to try and brighten her smile. I took one of the business cards that was on the counter's edge and proceeded to write a brief statement. I recalled a book of quotes my mother purchased for me when I was a kid, and I wrote on the back of the card: *If a man angers you, he conquers you. Pray!* I handed the card to her.

She looked up, surprised, and turned that frown into a big smile. "Thank you," she whispered.

"You're welcome." I grabbed the appointment papers she had for me and then turned and walked out, heading to my car and feeling pretty good about what I had just done.

I always believe in make people smile.

On the Friday of the same week, I left work in route to my general surgeon's office to meet with him regarding this biopsy thing that I was not very knowledgeable on. I was on time for my appointment. Since it is my first time there, I had to do the normal paperwork completion. There should be a standard doctor's document that serves as a cover to all doctors' visits so we don't have to keep filling out the same information repeatedly. After I completed the paperwork, I turned it in to the pleasant receptionist. I then sat back down on the nice comfortable couch to watch TV and/or thumb through the current magazines. I picked up a magazine to find an article to read. Before I could even get started, the nurse came and called out my name.

Well, how about that? I was getting my weight and vital measurements two minutes before my actual appointment time. There was a band playing songs of celebration in my head, and my thoughts were wrapped around the idea that I might get back to work in the time that I stated I would be back.

Quickly interrupted, the nurse asked me if I made the appointment or did my referring doctor. I told her that the doctor did. She stated that they had yet to receive my records from the referring doctor.

"I don't know why," I told her. "I am only following the instructions that were provided to me."

She said that she would continue to try and get in contact with the doctor's office while I met with the general surgeon. Unconcerned, I followed the nurse into the small patient's room and listened as she told me to sit on what looked like a high single bed with a thin paper sheet draped down the center of it. I hopped up on the electronic bed, and the nurse said the doctor would be in shortly.

As I waited, I looked around the office and saw the different posters that were related to the human breast, cancer stages, the human body's nerve layout, the 3D spinal and bone models, and the normal containers of gauze and Q-tips. I lay back as if I were going to get a nap, and just like when I visited my family doctor, the surgeon walked in before I could even close my eyes.

"Hello, Mr. Cameron, how are you?" he asked.

"I'm good," I replied.

He asked if my referring doctor knew that I was coming to see him.

"Of course he does," I responded, "because he made the appointment."

Eventually, the doctor brought the nurse in to ask if she got in contact with my doctor's office. She stated that they were not picking up the phone, so he told her to keep trying as we finished my appointment.

She said ok and left the room.

The surgeon began with an interview of my medical history before asking about what was currently going on.

I told him about an injury I received when I scraped my chest on the car door while working on the vehicle. Then there was the hit during a flag football game. I told him how I noticed the bruise, and how the knot under the bruise never went away after several weeks. I also told him that I had an ultrasound completed, which was the reason I was there now. They determined that there was a mass under my skin, and I needed to get it tested for any cancer cells. I also stated what my referring doctor told me about how a lot of men developed benign small tumors in the body. I guess that was my little way of seeing what his reaction would be to the information delivered to me.

He confirmed what the referring doctor had stated, and that confirmation brought a small level of satisfaction to me even though that satisfaction was not apparently visible in my body language. You know the social conception is that all of us men have to always appear calm and collected.

The surgeon explained what a biopsy was and how the day surgery would occur. On the day of surgery, I would be put under anesthesia, a small incision would be made at the location of the mass, and the mass would be extracted. They then would suture the wound and send me on my way. He said it would not take no time.

"OK," I said, "that would not be a problem."

We scheduled the surgery for the following week, and then he called the nurse back in to record the details. In the process of writing the details of the instructions, she stated she still could not get in contact with the doctor's office. I told them that I would try to call as well, but after repeated calls, I didn't get an answer.

"If I go and request the records, would it be beneficial that I get the records and bring them back?" I asked.

"It would definitely speed things up," the general surgeon replied. I could tell that the doctor was confused because he and the nurse were unable to get in contact with my family doctor. I decided to not go back to work immediately and instead to go to my family doctor to retrieve my records.

After I checked out with the receptionist, I called my family doctor again to no avail. As I drove to his office, I called again and finally got through. I told the lady on the other end that I was referred to a general surgeon, my family doctor made the appointment, but he did not send my records. I also stated that we needed the records for the general surgeon to review before we could proceed with the biopsy. Since the action to send the records to the surgeon had not been completed, I would be at their office in 15 minutes to pick up copies of my records.

When I got to the doctor's office, I walked into the crowded waiting room with a level of anger and disgust because I had to do their job while paying copays for an incomplete service. The lady at the front desk told me to go through the door that separated the waiting room from the medical area to speak with that receptionist. I proceeded through the door to get to the other receptionist. I told her that I called about my records, and I needed to pick them up. She said they were not quite ready.

"No problem," I said. "I will wait because my general surgeon needs them today, and I cannot leave just to come back."

After about 15 minutes of standing there waiting, people came out and checked out right next to me. In my mind, I was trying to be patient and respectable, but with each minute that passed, I made up my mind that I would not be coming back to this doctor. I was going to find me a new family doctor because this did not make sense. I could not continue to lose time with a doctor who did not genially care enough about his patients to have a supporting cast do their job with some high level of competence.

You try to support your community, and they continue to let you down. I had to be selfish with this situation and do what was best for me.

This is the last time, I thought.

I finally received my records, and I told the nurse, "Thank you."

When I returned the surgeon's office, which was on the other side of town from where my former family doctor's office resided, I walked in, and the general surgeon, the nurse that took my vitals, and the receptionist were all at the receptionist's desk. As gave them my records, I told them about what I had just gone through to get the records to them. They were looking with a sense of confusion, a look that seemed to say that this is the first time any patient had to go through such an effort. As I handed the records to the receptionist, the surgeon stated that he would review them, and if anything came up, he would let me know. Otherwise, he would see me the following week.

On January 6, 2010, I took off work for the day surgery. Since the doctor instructed me to take an additional day if possible, I went ahead and took off that Thursday and Friday as well. I had to be at the hospital at 6 a.m. for processing before my surgery that was scheduled for 8 a.m. I asked my mom to pick me up from my house at 5:30 a.m. so I could be on time. Now, I knew it was a 30-minute drive, but when I tell my mother a time, she always shows up 30 minutes early just to be on time. So, we left at approximately 5:15 a.m. I went in the hospital entrance and proceeded to the registration desk. I gave the lady my name, and she told me to fill out the stack of insurance and health papers. I handed the completed paperwork back to the receptionist, and she told me that they would be calling me in a few minutes. After about 10 minutes of waiting, they called me back to one of the registration rooms where a data entry associate confirmed all my information, copied my identification, and gave me your hospital identification band. The conversation was very light during this part of the process because we both were sleepy and needed a pick-me-up. She needed coffee, and I needed to be back in my bed. So, to help wake her and me up, I started telling situational jokes in my normal personable way. They also helped to make the time go by faster.

Now that I had received my arm band and was in the system for my procedure, I went to the large waiting room to wait to have my procedure. While there, I watched the little old school 27-inch TV that was in the large oversized media cabinet. Picture with me, it is 2009, and this hospital that charges $8 for one Tylenol pill cannot afford to get a larger flat screen TV for the waiting room. That TV definitely still utilized tubes. It reminded me of when we had the old small screen TV that had the two knobs in the 1980s when I was a little kid. You had to put the top number on channel 3 and rotate the lower knob to the many channels that it had. There were like 60 positions on the bottom knob as opposed to the 12 or so on the top knob. When the bottom knob broke off, we had to use a pair of pliers to change the channel. I also remember the antenna (also known as bunny ears) often having aluminum foil on the ends to help the reception come in better. I was in the waiting room thinking, *It is 2009, and they will not upgrade the TV.*

Oh well, at least the TV was color.

I heard my name called, and I got up and headed toward the greeter's desk.

I told them who I was, and the nurse asked, "Hi, are you ready?"

"Yes," I replied.

We went back to the day surgery area, and they showed me to my temporary bedding area. It was a cold room that had multiple bed stations where each station had its own hanging curtain that could be pulled around the bed for visual privacy. Please note that even though people could not see you, they definitely could still hear you. This means, please use your secret voice when you don't want others to hear what you have to say—especially if you may be embarrassed by what might be said.

So, as I pulled my clothes off and put on the gown that had the back end open, I remember thinking that they needed to do something to close those gowns up. Surely, we could get some oversized shirts or something. I put all my clothes and shoes in the little bag and lay down on the bed. After a few minutes, the nurse came in and asked if I would like a warm blanket.

"Yes, ma'am, I would," I replied.

When she brought the blanket and draped it over me, it reminded me of being a kid at my grandparents' south Alabama farm during the winters. My grandparents did not have centralized heat, so they used the fireplace to heat parts of the house. I remember blankets and quilts hanging in the doorways exiting the room where the fireplace was. This was so that the heat could be contained. We had to put more clothes on to move throughout the house. I recall that when I took a bath and put on my pajamas, I would go to the front room where most of the family would congregate around the fireplace. My mother would hold a blanket up to the fire for like two minutes. She would then wrap me in the blanket, and I would run and go jump in the bed. It felt like a warm hugging bear was squeezing me. During the night, you did not move because it would be so cold. This was a familiar feel in that cold hospital room with a warm blanket on me.

The nurse that wheeled me back and the anesthesiologist came behind the curtain to get my information to make sure they had the right patient and to start my IV. Now, I would be remiss if I did not acknowledge how cute the nurse was. I immediately started flirting with my eyes and that lip-biting smile. After all my information was obtained, they began to roll me back. As we were going back, we proceeded through all these heavy double doors. As we passed through each double door, it seemed like the lights were getting brighter. We finally got to the operating room that I would be going into. I remember thinking that it was seriously bright and cold in there. Besides that, I was happy to feel like everything was sterile and clean throughout the entire room. There were two other persons in the room already wearing the facial mask preparing the instruments and machines for the procedure. Playing in the background was some upbeat music. I nodded my head to the beat and asked the nurse pushing the bed were we getting ready to have a party? The people in the room started to chuckle.

She moved the rolling bed next to the operating table and let down the side rail attached to the bed. She then asked if I could hop onto the table.

"I sure can," I replied.

After sliding onto the operating table, they started putting straps across my arms and legs. Once the anesthesiologist came in, he had a brief conversation with the nurse that pushed me in.

"Now, we are going to give you a little gas to put you under," he said, "so what we need you to do is to take deep breaths when we put the mask on."

"That will not be a problem," I replied.

They put the mask on, and he said, "Ok, I am turning on the gas, so I will tell you when to take deep breaths."

I looked him in his eyes and nodded again. When he told me to start taking those deep breaths, I proceeded. After the first deep breath and exhale, nothing happened. With the second deep breath I took, again, nothing happened. On the third deep breath, I felt like I was becoming lightheaded. By the fourth deep breath, my eyes became really heavy, and my vision was blurry in a matter of a couple of seconds. On the fifth deep breath, I could barely open my eyes, and it felt like my body was a brick.

Then I remembered somebody calling my name repeatedly. I could hear them, but I could not open my eyes quickly. I had to work to get my eyes open. Then I finally got my eyes opened, and I felt very drunk. Now, I don't drink, but I imagine this was like a drunk's sensation. I tried to speak, but my voice was not working. I could not form any words or thoughts. It was a very funny yet helpless feeling. However, once you are fully up and out of the sleep sensation, you feel like you have just had the best rest a person could get in a 12-hour period. Although the surgery did not take but 20-30 minutes, it felt like I was asleep for half a day.

I finally came to my full senses, but I felt a little groggy still.

My mother was looking at me. "How you feel?" I asked.

"I am hungry and thirsty," I responded.

"Let me get the nurse. She might get you some ice."

After my mother returned, the nurse soon followed and had a cup of ice in her hand. She told me that everything went well and that the doctor would be in contact with me with my results. "When you're ready," the nurse began, "you can put your clothes on, and they will roll you out in a wheelchair to be discharged."

My mother left to retrieve the car and pull it up to the back door of the hospital where patients were discharged. I put my clothes on and waited for the nurse to get back with the wheelchair. When she did, she grabbed me by the arm to make sure I was stable when I stood from the bed. I sat down in the wheelchair.

"You will feel groggy for a while," she said. "You can have soup, but try not to eat heavy for a couple of hours."

As we got outside and rolled up to the car, I told the nurse, "Thank you."

"You're welcome." After she helped me get in the car, she added. "Get some rest."

I waved at her, and she waved back as we pulled off.

This entire situation was a crazy process. I had to do the work that my family physician should have been doing. I had worked through all these small situations just to have a surgery for what I expected to be routine tests. I am of the belief that the medical industry is out to make as much money as they can by ordering as many tests as possible. Now, it was just a waiting game before I would receive the test results—results that I believed would be negative.

CHAPTER 3 | THE BAD NEWS

On Monday, January 11, 2010, a week after having my biopsy, I was at work when I received a phone call from the general surgeon's nurse.

"We have received your test results," she said, "and the doctor would like for you to come in. What is the best time for you?"

"I can come in later today."

I prepared myself to go in because I knew there was something wrong with the diagnosis, but I figured it was a minor thing like I would probably have to take some medicine for some period of time.

That afternoon, I took a late lunch to go to the doctor. I figured I would pick something up on the way back to the office. While traveling to the doctor's office, I still thought that I this would be another routine for the medical industry to prescribe more medication to help sustain the multibillion-dollar industry.

I drove to the general surgeon's office thinking, *I rebuke anything that is against good health. I claim good health in the name of Jesus.* "This will not be anything big," I told myself. "Just another small issue that needs attention."

The receptionist was so welcoming when I entered the doctor's office. I told her my name and that I had an appointment. She said that she could see that I had an appointment and to have a seat before they called me back.

I went over to the sofa, picked up a magazine, and started flipping through the pages. The lady came to the door and called my name. I got up and proceeded to the scale that was sitting in the corner of the hallway. I got my weight reading and proceeded to the small room to the right down the hallway so I could take my vitals. After taking my vitals, the nurse showed me into the same small room that I had been going to since I had been coming to this general surgeon.

"The doctor will be in shortly," she said.

I remember sitting on the raised observation table thinking that I had to get back to work because I had a document that needed to be finished so I could submit it to editing as soon as possible. I was looking at the little spine model when the door opened.

The head nurse walked in first and smiled and said hello.

"Hello," I responded. "How are you?"

As she said, "I am doing good," the general surgeon walked in about three paces behind her and said, "Hello, how are you doing?" As he was completing his question, he turned and reached behind him to close the door.

"I am well," I answered.

"That's good." As he looked down the clipboard in his hand, the next thing out of his mouth was, "Well, I have some bad news. It appears that you have cancer."

I looked at him, knowing that I heard what he said, but it did not register right then what he had said. I looked him in his eye with a slight facial shrug with my left eyebrow up, and that had the corner of my mouth slightly in grin.

In a calm voice, I said to him, "Cancer?"

"Yes, breast cancer."

I looked immediately to the floor as I was processing what he said. How could I possibly have breast cancer? Men do not get breast cancer. In a mere second after looking at the floor, I felt my heart sink down to my stomach. I could only imagine what I looked like at that moment. I remember thinking how could this happen to me. What have I done to deserve this? My eyes took in the general surgeon, and with despair in my voice, I asked, "How long do I have to live?"

"All we know now is that you have cancer growing in my body."

He left my right side where he delivered the news and proceeded to walk between me and the nurse to point to the poster/chart of cancer stages, which was on the wall to my immediate left. The poster explained the human breast and how the nerves and ducts operate in the breast. On that poster was a chart explaining the stages of cancer. He explained that my tumor had grown to approximately 2 cm in diameter, which means I was at stage two. On the poster that he was using to explain, he pointed to the area that showed tumor sizes and the relative stage of cancer they represent.

"Could this happen?" I asked. "Do men get breast cancer?"

"Men do get it, but it is not in as high frequency as it is in women."

As he walked back to his position on my right side, where he stood between the nurse and the door, I really started processing that I could be dying, and I started to tear up. I tried my best to be strong and not show any emotions, but the more thoughts that passed through my head in the three or four seconds it took for him to get back to his position, the harder it became.

I thought about my mother—what would she do if I died? This devastating news could kill her. What about my daughter? She would never get the chance to know the full capacity of who I am. What kind of legacy would I leave her? Who would make sure she stayed on the right path? What about my lady? We had started making big plans. How was she going to take this news? What about the rest of my family and friends? Did this mean I was less than a man? What was wrong with me? Was there something wrong with my DNA? Was I prone to diseases as I got older?

The tears came down my face. I know my eyes had to have been red. I remember finally looking at the nurse's eyes, and she had this look that I will never forget. Her look of devastation was so great that I felt like she was my mother with a heartfelt virtual cry ringing through the atmosphere. She began tearing up as she turned and reached for the box of tissue. As she picked up the box and handed it to me, I pulled about three tissue sheets out. When she pulled it back, she took a few for herself and began wiping her tears as well.

"What are the next steps that I have to take?" I asked the surgeon.

He recommended that I have a mastectomy on my left breast.

When I asked him, "What is that?" he explained that it was the removal of the nipple, glands, and fat tissue that make up the breast.

"That's the complete removal of the left breast?" How would this make it look? I had wondered.

He further explained that a part of the muscle would have to be removed and that part of the chest would be flat and just have a scar.

"You mean that I would only have one nipple?" When he answered yes, in a vain moment, I asked, "What about my other breast?"

"In some cases," he began, "the cancer can return in the other breast later."

"What do you recommend I do?"

He replied that if it were him, he would go ahead and remove both to reduce the chances of the tumor returning.

"So that means you would completely remove both breasts?"

"Yes."

This was crazy. What would I look like? How would I move forward in life? The more we continued to talk, the more I tried to process. As an engineer, I was taught critical thinking. I was trying to process and solve this problem in real time. I was trying to navigate my questions to retrieve more information while processing the fact that my life was on limited time.

"How fast do we need to move on this?" I asked.

"Given the stage your cancer is in, we need to move fairly quickly." He added that he could probably get me in that same week.

The nurse began looking on the laptop that she was holding for dates. She gave me options for date and time combinations. I chose Thursday, January 14, 2010.

My composure slowly returned. "What's the next step regarding the cancer?" I asked.

He told me that I needed to find an oncologist, and I told him that I wanted to use Dr. Paul Dang. I got Dr. Dang's name from Mr. Lloyd Brooks, my former program manager (PM) on a contract that we were working on together. When I met

Lloyd, he was going through chemotherapy for Leukemia. He and the company's human resources manager interviewed me at the Embassy Suites. I had been talking to the HR manager regarding the position, so the Embassy Suite interview gave me my unknowingly strong relationship beginning with Lloyd. Lloyd was hairless all over his head and wasn't feeling good. At times, he would have to get up and excuse himself from the interview. I was the first engineer that Lloyd hired for the new contract.

From my hiring to the time Lloyd decided to step down as the PM of the contract, we talked about his family history with cancer and his choice in Dr. Dang. It was those conversations with Lloyd that had me ready with a name of an oncologist. Mr. Brooks warned me about the effects of chemical therapy, such as the skin turning a much darker shade, nail color changes, sickness, low immune system, nausea, and random side effects. It is funny how God will know what you need before you have any clue of what you are going to have to go through; therefore, the provisions that you need are provided right on time.

After I informed Dr. Fernandez whom I chose to be my oncologist, he stated that he knew of Dr. Dang, and he was a well-respected doctor. He then stated that his office would help me set up an appointment to see Dr. Dang. He summarized my preparation for surgery and told me that they would be sending the detailed information home with me.

I followed the nurse to the front receptionist. Seeing a few people sitting in the lobby, I tried to keep my back turned to them while I received my information. The nurse stood behind the receptionist, staring at me as I got my papers.

As I turned to leave, she said, "Good Luck, Mr. Cameron. Have a good day."

With a slight crackle in my voice, I said, "Thank you," and turned to walk out of the office.

The walk to my car was long. The two hallways before reaching the outside sliding doors seemed like walking the Green Mile. While I was walking, I thought, *I have to go tell my mother.*

I had no clue how she would take it. I did not know how I was going to take her response, but I had to be strong.

As I got to my car, I knew that I was not going back to work, and I did not even think about calling them to let them know that I would not be back. I took that company provided BlackBerry and sent an email to those in need of knowing that I would not be returning for the rest of the day. I remember getting into the car and starting it. Before I could even put on my seatbelt, I broke down crying. I could be in my last days, I thought. I had so many dreams accomplished with so many more to achieve. *Why is God punishing me? What have I done?*

I cried hard; it was as if I had received one of those early childhood whoopings when I did something I had no business doing. The kind of crying that you pause in the middle of to take that hard gasp for air only to repeat the cycle because your heart is in such despair.

After a couple of minutes of crying and saying aloud, "Lord, help me," I started to gain my composure. Although the tears continue to stroll down my face, I began to drive to my mother's home on the other side of town. I thought about having to tell her and tell the woman I was talking to at the time.

In the middle of my travel to my mother's home, my lady friend text me and asked me what the doctor said. I did not know how to respond, so I texted her that I was just leaving the doctor and would call her when I got back. I knew she would pick up that something was wrong, but I was hoping that I could soften the blow by talking to instead of texting her. Now, my stress level increased even more as I drove. With every second driving, the weight of my heart increased tenfold as I got closer to my mom's home.

Pulling up in her yard, I told myself, "You have to pull yourself together." I tried to wipe my face and take multiple deep breaths so I could be calm when I walked in.

I got out of the car and walked up to the door and rang the doorbell. I looked up to the sky and remember seeing the clouds scrolling across the blue background while the wind breezed across my eyebrows, slightly drying the tears that settled there.

My mom opened the inner door first, then the security door. "Hey, how is it going?" she asked.

I looked down when I stepped past her while saying, "Good."

I walked to the middle of the living room and turned back to her as she closed the doors. She looked at me, and as I looked her in her eyes, I teared up and said, "I have cancer."

The look on her face was something that I wished I could forget. She frowned and began to tear up. She opened her arms and walked toward me to embrace me. I walked to her and began to cry again. We stood there, embracing each other in a moment of displaying the greatest thing about living in this world–LOVE.

As she held and squeezed me, she said, "It will be ok, Derrick. God is in control. He did not bring you this far to let you down now. He has a plan for you, and your work is not done. You have to keep the faith. We are going to get through this, too."

At that very moment, Mother prayed with and for me. "You have to calm down," she said before releasing her hold from me and walking over to the wall piece that she got while we were in Germany.

She retrieved her blessed oil. As she returned to me, she put some oil in her hand. "Lift up your shirt," she said.

As I lifted my shirt, she sat the bottle down and began to rub her hands together. Then, she began to pray and rub the oil on my chest. I closed my eyes and prayed along with her. A sense of calm came over me. Months later, my mother told me what she experienced in that moment. When she got the oil and prayed over me while applying the oil, her hand became burning hot. This was not heat from friction nor was it from a chemical in the oil to make it hot. The heat was the evil spirit leaving the body.

After praying over me, she asked if I wanted something to drink. I said yes. I took that opportunity to text my lady, telling her to call me when she got a chance. Within a minute, she called me.

I started our talk with the typical *Hi, how are you* chatter, but she got right to the point, asking, "What did the doctor say?"

I took a deep breath. "I have cancer."

"Really?"

"Yes."

"Where are you now?" she asked.

I told her I was over my mom's house, and she replied she'd be there in a minute. Knowing it would take her about 10 minutes to get there, I took that time to sit down and get my composure together. I would definitely have to be strong for her. To calm myself, I drank the water my mom had fixed and meditated while sitting in the living room that faced the driveway.

When my lady pulled up, I could see her through the sheer curtains. She walked up and rang the doorbell. As soon as I opened the doors, she walked in, looked at me, and began crying. As I embraced her, I realized the level of our Love. She was crying hard, and I told her everything would be ok. We stood there for a couple of minutes holding each other. I finally loosened my embrace to close the door. In that time, my mother came in and hugged her as well.

"Everything will be ok," Mom told her before returning to the kitchen.

I took my lady's hand and led her to the couch in the living room so we could sit. She rested her head on my shoulder while she put the back of her left hand, which was clutching a tissue, on my right thigh. We sat there for a while just talking about what the doctor said and what the upcoming plans were for the operation. I explained everything I knew to her. She began crying again, and I echoed my mother's sentiment: "Everything will be ok."

In a stressed voiced, she said, "I don't want to lose you."

"You will never lose me. I am always in your heart, but you won't lose me on this earth either because I have a fight to win."

We remained entwined on the couch for a while longer until she had to leave. I hugged and kissed her goodbye, and I told her that she had to calm down. Everything would be ok.

As she walked to her vehicle, I said, "Remember that I love you."

"I love you, too," she said.

"Now let me see you smile." With a little effort, she did. "I want to see some teeth."

Giggling, she said, "You play too much."

"No," I replied, "I love too much. I will talk to you later."

It is amazing how the person you are in love with can make a seemingly impossible situation seem like a minor bump in the highway.

After she left, I told my mom I had to go lay down for a minute because I was exhausted. While resting, I thought about so many things, like life, being scared, and wondering what would cause me or what would cause God to inflate this kind of pain and disease on me. Eventually, I fell into a short sleep, and as I woke up, just as clear as day, a thought came through my mind like a clear voice, "Let it beat you, or you can beat it." So, I decided to either get busy living or to get busy dying. I was not going to let this disease beat me or at least not without a fight. So, from that point forward, I realized it was time for me to focus and understand what I was facing. I had to keep a positive attitude and be proactive instead of reactive. I had to remove any known or perceived negative entities from my life. Some of those negative forces are your family members. It is ok to separate yourself from consistent negativity.

It was time for a new chapter in my life, and I had to be focused on getting through this chapter as best as I could.

Unknowingly, while I was meditating on my situation, my mother was packing her clothes to come over to my house to be with me that night and for several nights thereafter. I went home to start getting ready for my upcoming procedures and get everything in order. Approximately an hour or two after getting home, my mother called me and said open the garage. When she walked in, she had a bag with her. What I thought would be a few days of staying with me turned into an extended stay. She had committed herself to walking with me through every step of what would be coming.

On Thursday, January 14, 2010, I was scheduled to have my double mastectomy. I could not even sleep the night before. I had awakened and lain there in the dark for a little while looking at the ceiling. I was wondering how all this could be happening so fast, how I was about to forever alter my body physically. It was amazing how I really didn't worry about my physical appearance before the surgery, other than the small things like needing to work on my forearms to even out my arms. Now I was staring in the mirror thinking that this was the last time I would have nipples. As I thought about the uncertainty of the surgery, I rubbed my hand across my chest a few times.

Then I said to myself, "Well, let's get it!"

My mother was already up and sitting at the kitchen table as I walked up to the kitchen from the back. She was reading her bible and asked was I ready when I walked into the kitchen.

"Yes, I am," I replied. "Let's get this over with." So, we departed and headed for the hospital.

When we arrived, my mother and I went to the check-in area and then the waiting area. While there, I saw my good friend Tasha and one of my mentors, Mr. Young. I also noticed my pastor on the opposite side of the room. I spoke to Tasha and gave her a hug. I then spoke to my mentor, and while I was sitting down, one of my mother's friends came in. We all went to the side my pastor was on to pray. My mentor prayed, then my pastor, and finally my mom. After the prayer, we all went to the far side of the waiting room to take our seats, excluding my pastor who had to go visit another person from the church. While waiting, two of my motorcycle buddies, BJ and Marlon, came in. I expected both of them because BJ told me they were coming to the hospital when he came by the house the night before with our mutual buddy Vince.

The night before, BJ and Vince came by after learning the news that I had cancer. My boys, whom I have known since college, came to show support. The conversation was light as we remembered past adventures together. We danced around the topic for a while before the conversation died down and that awkward silence filled the room. Finally, one of them asked the question: how did this come to happen.

I told them how I found it and what had occurred up to that day. A look of great sadness was on their faces; it was as if they thought, *One of three amigos could actually be dying.* None of us really understood what this disease was or what it took to fight it. We sat there talking until about 1 a.m. until BJ said, "Man, we need to get up so you can get your rest."

"All right, bro."

As we got up from where we were sitting, I looked each of them in the eye and said, "I'll be all right."

We walked to the front door, and as they were leaving out, I gave both of them that half handshake, half hug.

"All right, dude," he said. "We will see you tomorrow." Watching them leave, I knew that the bond among me, Vince, and BJ was strengthened that night.

While we waited for me to be called back for my procedure, there were a lot of side conversations going on. I was checking my phone, responding to text messages. My lady was texting me that she had just got to the hospital. I told her where she would fine us, and as she walked in, she spotted me and started walking toward us. My mother saw her coming and told her friend to move over so my lady could sit next to me. This action caught the attention of everyone because they had never met my lady before.

As she came close, I got up and gave her a hug then we sat down. While sitting there having our low playful conversation, I stroked her hands in an effort to keep her calm. It was good to have so many people there when I was going through my new challenge. I never thought that so many people loved and cared about me to this extent.

After my extended wait in the waiting room, they finally called my name to go to the pre-operation area. I briefly squeezed my lady's hand and told everyone, "Well, here we go."

Personnel told me that once I was prepared for surgery, they would let a couple of family members come back. I followed the nurse back to the pre-operation area, and she went through the same routine as before: giving me a surgical gown to put on and telling me to take off everything but my underwear and socks. After I took my clothes off, I put them in the plastic bag that was provided and lay on the cold bed.

She came back in and said that she had to get some information. As she started asking me what seemed like 100 questions, another nurse came in and said she was going to get the IV started. Several questions and a couple of needle pokes later, I was ready for surgery. They called for family to come back.

After a few minutes, my mother and my lady came to see me. I was telling jokes to lighten the mood and to keep my lady entertained. I could tell she was concerned by the entire situation. When the anesthesiologist and the nurse came in and gave me information about the procedure, I recognized the nurse. It was Alicia, the woman whom one of my former motorcycle club members was dating and would eventually marry. It turned out she had assisted in my mom's eye surgery. I was a little relieved to know someone who would be in there with me. I guess we officially had a family nurse now.

"Let's say a quick prayer," my mom said.

Everyone bowed, and I closed my eyes as my mom said a brief prayer for the procedure. When she completed, she looked at me as if she was saying you got this. I looked at my lady and reached out for her. She took my hand, and I told her, "You better give me a kiss. You know I need the luscious before I go in here." She kissed me on the lips. "Don't you feel better?"

She laughed while shaking her head. "You and your kissing self."

I chuckled as they began to roll me to the back. The atmosphere was the same as before–music playing in the operating room, me grooving to the music when we got back there in that cold room. I saw Alicia and two more individuals in there preparing for surgery. Alicia rolled me next to the operating table and told me to hop over to the other table. After I hopped up on the table, she started to strap me onto it. By that time, Dr. Fernandez came in. He asked me how I was doing? I said fine.

I was still telling jokes. I made the statement, "Since you are taking off my chest, do you mind taking a little off the sides and front? I have to let my six pack in this cooler show." Everyone in the operating room laughed. I looked at the surgeon and added, "Why are you laughing? I mean you already going to be cutting. Won't you hook me up?" I was only encouraging the chuckles from everyone. By then, the anesthesiologist told me he was going to put something in my IV to make me feel good first, and then he was going to put the medicine in the IV. I would feel lightheaded at first, and then my eyes would feel heavy, and then, I would be waking up post-surgery.

Well, it happened just like that because the next thing I remember was waking up in the recovery room.

As I regained my awareness, I remember waking up under a blanket. The nurse told me to be careful because I had two tubes coming out of my chest for draining.

I looked at her perplexed because I had no idea of what she was talking about. "Really?"

"Yes."

I lifted up the blanket and saw the bandages across my chest and a clear tube coming out of each side of my chest right at the level that my nipples used to be. The tubes were at the ends of two horizontal cuts that were about six inches long and ended just before the armpit. I could not really see what was going on under the bandages, but I could see that these clear tubes had what looked like blood residue in the tubes. The nurse told me that they had to put the tubes in my chest for drainage of excess fluid after the surgery. After a while, the surgeon came in and told me that I would have to wear the drain tubes for about two weeks.

Having the drainage bags was an interesting time. I would have to drain the tubes at least once a day and then record how much drainage came from each side of my chest on a daily basis. It was amazing to see science at work. The fluid that built up in my chest would drain through the tubes and collect in the hard plastic containers attached at the end of the tubes. The containers had tops that could screw off for easy liquid disposal. I would usually wear an undershirt to hold the tubes close to the skin while I would attach each collecting container on my waistband or my belt when wearing slacks. When I finally went back to work and was wearing the drainage containers, I would usually wear a casual jacket with my ensemble so it would hide the tubes attached to my belt.

After having to wear the drainage containers for several weeks, I had the tubes taken out. I was sitting on the table waiting on the doctor and the nurse to extract the tubes. I wasn't sure what to expect. I was a little eager to see what was about to happen. After the doctor and nurse put on the latex gloves, he asked me if I was ready to get the tubes removed. After I replied yes, he gently put one hand at the center of my chest and started to slowly tug on one tube with the other hand. He slowly pulled the tube from under the skin, which felt a little weird. It felt as if my skin was a little numb. After removing the tube, he then got a Band-Aid and placed it over the incision. He immediately did the opposite side the same way and sent me on my way. He told me to monitor my chest, and if I had any issues to come back to see him. I initially thought that I was good when I left, unaware that I would be coming back about a week later.

In the time that initially passed after removing the drainage tubes, everything seemed to be ok. Then in some days, I started to feel like I was losing my breath, as if an elephant was standing on my chest. In addition to the shortness of breath, it seemed like I kept hearing a swishing noise but was not certain what it was. About the fourth day from after having the tubes removed, I was in the shower and noticed my chest was puffy like it was starting to swell. As I would push on my chest with my index finger, I noticed that it felt like fluid was under the skin. That is when I knew that fluid was building on my chest. I immediately called the doctor, but he was away on vacation, so I was referred to another doctor that was seeing Dr. Fernandez's patients while he was away.

While I was talking to the nurse at the referring doctor's office, she asked me some questions and told me that I should come in that same day. I put on some clothes and proceeded to head down to the referring doctor's office. When I walked in, I thought I was in a movie. The scene that I had walked into looked like a free clinic where some doctor was providing free health care to anyone one for a limited time in the day. There were so many people there for so many different things. People were there of all ages, young mothers with babies crying and older couples waiting to see the doctor. We were all stuffed in a small waiting room like we were sardines in a can. After about two hours, the doctor finally worked me in, and I went back to one of the patients' rooms. I told him who my surgical doctor was and why I was there. When I told him that I had breast cancer, he looked surprised. He wanted me to confirm that he heard me right. "Yes," I told him, "I am a breast cancer survivor." He then asked how I found the cancerous tumor. He seemed more enthusiastic about my story, but he quickly remembered that he did not have a lot of time to explore how I got to be there.

He asked me to lift up my shirt and lay back. As I was laying on the platform, he started to feel on and around my pectoral. "Yes," he said, "you have fluid on your chest, so we are going to have to drain it."

I became a little nervous because I wasn't sure how this was going to get accomplished, so I asked him how he was going to drain the liquid. He told me that he and his assistant would drain the liquid using syringes. He asked the nurse to get some syringes. I was thinking she was going to get a couple of those small syringes they use to get blood with. The nurse came back with large syringes that were about 1 inch in diameter and about 6 inches long. The needle itself looked as if it was about 3 inches long and about as wide as a sewing needle.

The doctor removed both Band-Aids and handed his assistant a syringe. He proceeded to insert the syringe in my right pectoral incision and start slowly pulling back on the syringe plunger. I noticed the liquid starting to be collected in the huge clear syringe. The assistant soon followed the doctor's actions on my chest's left side. Everything was going ok at first until it seemed that they had to move the needle around under my skin to make sure that they got as much of the liquid as possible. They started swiping the needles back and forward, which produced a very intense stinging sensation. I almost jumped up off the table, but I had to be still so I did not inject the needle into any vital organs.

This process lasted for several minutes but felt like an eternity. The doctor filled one and a half syringes from the right side of my chest. The assistant filled one full syringe and a quarter of another large syringe. After they were done collecting as much liquid as possible, they removed the syringes and placed Band-Aides back on my entry points. I immediately felt relief from the painful chest exploration as I could take a deep breath. For some time after all of the complications, I would have what I call "ghost itching" in my chest. It felt like my nipples would be itching, and when I went to scratch them, they would not be there. So, I would rub my chest in an effort to subdue the itching. This happened for an extended period of time.

With the surgery completed, I wanted to make sure I helped my body deal with the chemical therapy treatment. I did some light research about the human body. The truth of the matter is that the body is a self-sustaining mechanism. People survived for hundreds of years without current medicine available. I have always been aware of how people of prior generations lived healthier and longer lives. Earlier generations were far more mobile and ate far healthier. I knew I had to change my way of living, especially during this time. My diet had to change, and my exercise routine would take a setback. But to help my body become more effective in dealing with the chemical treatment that I had reluctantly agreed to, I decided to frequently visit a chiropractor to help make sure my central nervous system was tuned to its best.

I read studies on how people have scientifically healed without manufactured medicines. These individuals would practice natural herb healing. I believed that natural herbal medication would give my body every opportunity to react positively to the upcoming invasive chemical as well as give me every opportunity to rest well at night. I visited Huntsville Chiropractic twice a month. Every visit was an inspirational visit. The staff was so nice, and they made me feel at home. It was not long before they knew me by name and knew my story. It was not long before they gave me a nickname. Visiting the chiropractor was a great decision because I could definitely feel tension release immediately, and I slept better most nights. The benefits from getting my spine worked were immediate. I felt that as long as I sustained my visits to the chiropractor I would be physically ready to endure what was to come. Now it was time to meet my oncologist for the first time.

CHAPTER 4 | CHEMOTHERAPY AND MAINTAINING MY LIFESTYLE

I went to Crestwood Hospital to meet Dr. Paul Dang for the first time, and my mother decided to join me. When we arrived at the Cancer Institute section on the third floor, I checked in, not knowing what to expect. However, Dr. Dang seemed very nice. He asked me how I had found my lump, and I told him about finding it in the shower. I also told him about when I scraped my chest against the door of the car that I was working over. I was curious if there was any chance that when I scraped my left breast on the door, that caused me to get cancer. He said that it was highly unlikely.

Before we started talking about all of my options, Dr. Dang wanted to see the results of my surgery, so he asked me to lift up my shirt. When he inspected the wounds and saw where the scabs were forming from the drain tubes that were installed in my chest, he asked me how much discharge I was receiving daily. When I told him, he stated that the amount was about what he would expect.

Dr. Dang had been reviewing my files and my blood work and stated that I probably developed the breast cancer from having increased estrogen levels. The moment I heard that, I began thinking all sorts of things; I didn't know what that meant. Mr. Dang had to explain to me that everyone has testosterone and estrogen levels. The idea is to keep the right balance in the body. My immediate concern became how did my levels become unbalanced.

He proceeded to tell me what all of my options were. He said chemotherapy was a choice that I had, but it would not be necessary. I could choose to take the chemotherapy to help reduce the possibility of the cancer returning. What he would do was cut down on the percentage of any cancer cells being in the body as well as prevent it from coming back. I had a choice to either do 12 chemotherapy sessions or 16 sessions. I asked him what the probability was that the cancer would not return if I chose 12 sessions versus 16 sessions. He told me that there was about a 28% chance of the cancer returning if I didn't take chemotherapy. There was about a 20% chance of the cancer returning if I only did 12 sessions, and there was about a 12% chance if I did 16 sessions. These numbers were approximation to the effects of taking chemotherapy. I decided to go with the 16 sessions because he stated that I was young and strong enough to handle the medicine with the hope that I would have little side effects. He did not offer information on stem cell treatment; however, I inquired about it.

After receiving the information about stem cell research, I decided to stick with chemotherapy, so Dr. Dang stated there were simple medicines that I would have to take, and he would provide information such as cost and side effects on each medication. He also informed me that it was a possibility that I would become unable to have kids. Therefore, there was an option for me to freeze my sperm at a sperm bank just in case I became sterile and could not have more kids. He gave me information and the contact information for the sperm bank, so I could contact them on what the procedure would be and how much it would cost. I figured that I would call the sperm bank and get the information on freezing sperm. I would need to determine pretty quickly if I would either freeze my sperm, which could take up to two weeks to make sure that plenty of sperm was obtained, or immediately start my chemotherapy sessions.

Although I had all the information that I needed about the medicines, I still had questions about what chemotherapy would do to my sex life. I could not ask the doctor intimate questions while my mother was in the room. My plan was to call back the next day for a visit so I could ask how chemotherapy my affect intimacy. My mom and I left after I scheduled my next appointment, the one in which I would do blood work.

The next day, I called the sperm bank to get information on what it would take to freeze sperm, how much it would cost, and how long it would last. They told me that they would give me a special condom to use during sex, and I would have a certain amount of time—a couple of hours—to get the condom, after placing it in a special bag, back to them. They also gave me the option of coming in and using a private room at the facility to retrieve then provide them a specimen. Obviously, I didn't want to do the masturbation, so I decided that if I was going to freeze any sperm, then I would use my partner, but first I would have to talk to her about what she thought about it. I already knew that the answer would be just what it was, that it would not be a problem.

That same day, I went back to see the doctor to ask him about what chemotherapy would do to my sexual encounters. He told me that the biggest problem could be that I become sterile. There were no expected side effects to getting an erection. However, he suggested that I still use condoms for protected sex because "You don't want any of the medicine expunged into the sperm to be used to fertilize an egg."

In my days of deliberation, I really thought about my faith, and I believed that if it was meant for me to have any more kids, then God would be in control. So, I decided not to freeze any sperm and trust that God would deliver kids if it was within his will. With this decision made, the next goal was to start my chemotherapy as soon as possible. When I called Dr. Dang and told him of my decision, we made our first planned treatment for February 11, 2010.

Before my first treatment, I was scheduled to take a Computerized Axial Tomography (CAT) scan and a Positron Emission Tomography (PET) scan at CCI. The scans were used to determine a baseline for receiving the chemotherapy treatments and would be taken again during and post treatments. The night before, I could not eat anything and was instructed to drink only clear liquids for the scan. The CAT scan is used to take detailed pictures inside the body whereas a PET scan helps determine the exact location of the cancer inside the body. The PET scan is the one that doesn't sound too biologically friendly. A PET scan requires the use of a radioactive substance to be injected into the patient's vein. According to some research I did on www.cancer.net, the substance is absorbed mainly by organs and tissues that use the most energy and then depicted in the scan as the organs and tissue in the body. This procedure takes a few hours. I remember going into a room with only a chair when I went to get my PET scan. They put you in a recliner, inject this die in your arm, then they will tell you to be still as much as possible for more than an hour. I remember the nurse gave me a blanket and turned the lights to dim and said feel free to fall asleep. I took her up on the offer and went to sleep. I really did not move once I was in the reclined position. After about an hour, the nurse returned and led me to the scanning area. Once again, they asked me to not move a muscle so they could get a good scan. The scan took approximately 30–45 minutes, and during that time, the machine took about 5-7 different scans while I lay motionless on the table. For each scan, I was inserted into the machine via an electronic sliding table. The machine was not loud like that of an MRI machine.

The CAT and PET scan experiences at CCI were much more pleasant compared to when I went to get a PET scan at another location. At the previous scan, I was stuck in about 10 locations with this needle filled with die. It first felt like a wasp sting that would increasingly get painful like someone was taking the tip of a knife to try to dig out a splinter from your chest. This sensation would occur in every insertion of the dye filled syringe. I remember looking at the nurse, and she said, "You are definitely a trooper because you are not saying anything."

I told her it still hurt.

"I've had grown men come up off the table, and I had to move the needle before they impaled themselves deeply." She also told me that sometimes she had to stick people in between all of their toes. That statement there made my stomach ball into a knot. I could only imagine taking that large needle in between my toes and then have her inject that dye. I could only shake my head. As bad as some of the scans would be, they were necessary to track the performance of the chemotherapy treatments.

My first chemotherapy session was done at Crestwood Hospital. When my mother and I arrived at the cancer center's receptionist area, I was given paperwork to fill out. As I looked at the papers, I thought, *I have no idea what I'm about to get myself into.* After completing what seemed like a book of paperwork, I returned the batch of papers back to the receptionist and sat there waiting for my name to be called in turn. I noticed a couple of people waiting along with me. A nurse came to the door leading to the back and called out a name for the next patient. She did this three or four times before calling my name. When I heard my name, a high level of anxiety came over me as I walked to the door.

"How are you doing?" she asked.

"I'm ok. How are you?"

She responded in kind and said she was doing good.

The door closed behind me somewhat hard, and it felt like I was going to lockdown.

The nurse took me to a small room with several chairs that had a single rotating arm. This was where people gave blood so that it could be checked before people proceeding to treatment.

I remember my general surgeon explained to me that during the double mastectomy, he had pulled the lymph nodes from under my left arm to do a quick test for any cancer cells that might had traveled to the lymph nodes. The test was negative, and they reinserted the lymph nodes before sewing me back up. The surgeon also explained that the lymph node test would restrict me from having my blood pressure checked or blood drawn from my left arm, so I told the technician that was to take my blood that he would have to pull the blood from my right arm.

So, all of my visits routinely became a check-in, a technician asking me for my name and date of birth to verify that the four or five small tubes that needed to be filled with my blood were labeled with my name and information. The technician would then pull out the surgical rubber band and a butterfly clip style needle that retracted by a loaded spring when the edges were pushed down. I appreciated the ease of this new style of needle with the tube connector on the end over the use of the old needles to have your blood drawn. New technology is making our medical experiences a ton less stressful. You can pop one tube on the end of the butterfly needle, and as it fills up the airtight tube, you can pull the tube off once the right blood level is reached then replace it with another tube to collect more blood. Once done, you can retract the needle and have a nice and clean disposal.

After filling all the tubes of blood, they put the folded gauze on my arm then self-adhesive tape and told me to leave the gauze on for about 10 minutes. During that time, I walked down a small hallway to an area where they took my vitals (weight, blood pressure, and oxygen levels) while they confirmed all medicines that I had been taking.

A nurse's assistant put the blood pressure cuff on my right arm and began to take my pressure.

She looked at me and asked, "Is your blood pressure normally this high?"

"I don't know what is considered high," I replied, "but I am a little nervous about being here for the first time."

Nodding, she said, "Oh, that is understandable."

After doing a second blood pressure reading for a second time, the nurse saw my numbers drop a bit, so she wrote it down and then asked me to get up and step on the electronic scale to be weighed. Once my weight and medications were noted, I was told that my blood levels looked fine to proceed. This was the go-ahead moment to go get all the chemotherapy medicine ready while they led me to the treatment areas.

While walking, I saw a bunch of reclining chairs with an IV stand next to each chair and a volume control machine hooked about midway up the IV stand. There were two rows going east and west with about six chairs in a row. Imagine walking into an open room with two rows of chairs facing each other and an eight-foot aisle way between. There were about eight more chairs along the adjacent hallway.

As I walked in, every nurse was so nice and welcoming. One nurse led me to the chairs that were against the wall and told me to choose anywhere to sit. I picked the chair that was on the back wall so I could see people walking in and out. I wanted to see what traffic would be coming through while I was getting my treatment. When I sat, I noticed that it was cold in the room. They offered a blanket and something to drink like a little water or apple juice or orange juice. They also offered something to eat like crackers. Before they began the treatment, the doctor examined the blood analysis and my vital signs to see if and how to proceed with treatment. I remembered on one occasion before I could start, I had to lower my blood pressure by trying to relax. As I told the nurse, my blood pressure might had been up because of stress. After about a 45-minute delay, I was able to get my blood pressure down so we could begin.

The medicine they brought out had my identification on it, and again, they asked my name and date of birth to verify that I was who I said I was, and that I was getting the right medicine. I noticed the nurse also brought what looked like an oversized Ziploc bag with several large and small syringes. This would be the first time that I would see the steroids and the three main administered drugs–Doxorubicin Hydrochloride (Adriamycin), Cyclophosphamide (Cytoxan), and Taxol (paclitaxel). The bag also included smaller bags of medicine and the cleaning solution. They used this solution at the beginning, between the use of each medicine, and after the final medicine to thoroughly clean out the port by injecting it through the port.

I was nervous because I did not know what to expect. The nurse sat on a rolling stool and, once again, asked for information to verify that all the medicine in the bag belonged to me. She then proceeded to put on the blue surgical gloves and ask me which arm did I want to administer the medicine to. After telling her that I had a port put in my chest so I would not have to take the needles in the arm, she asked me to lift up my shirt so she could clean the port area. I took my left arm out of my sleeve so my shirt could drape around my neck. I watched as the nurse took out a cleaning pad that looked like a small wet nap and wiped the skin over the port. Before leaving the house that morning, I had put on a prescribed cream that was supposed to help numb the area around the port. The cream seemed to be working because I could barely feel the nurse's hands working around the port. When she pulled out the first needle to dispense the cleaning solution, she told me the name of the solution and what it was being used for.

The nurse inserted the needle in the top of the port about a quarter of an inch and then pushed the syringe's plunger slowly. After pushing all the solution into the port, she then picked up the next syringe and told me that this medicine would give me a bad taste in my mouth.

"Do you have a peppermint to suck on while I dispense the medicine?" she asked.

I looked at my mother and asked her if she had a piece of peppermint candy. She usually carried peppermints, and she did not disappoint me by not having a piece this day. I popped the piece of candy in my mouth, and the nurse said, "Ok, here we go."

Although I was eating the peppermint, I could still taste the medicine while it was being dispensed in the port. The taste was like I was eating metal. I had never tried eating metal before, but I promise I feel like I know what metal tastes like. The taste stays with you several minutes after the first time you receive the medicine. After all the liquid had been dispensed from the syringe, the nurse then removed it and picked up another syringe filled with the cleaning solution.

The next medicine to be administered, the steroid, also had a very weird effect on me. The nurse warned me that the medicine could make me feel like I had ants in my pants. I smirked when she said it because I thought she was playing. Several seconds after she began administering the medicine, it really did feel like I had ants in my pants, crawling under the skin of my inner thighs. Later, I would find out that the faster you administer this medicine, the more active the sensation increases. I did come to find out that the steroids would make me constipated. The doctor warned me that this could happen and offered yet another prescription for medication that would counter the side effects of the steroids. The subscription would not be needed as I would find out later that if you take a high dosage of vitamin C daily, you will have loose-bowel movements. After the dosage of steroids was administered, the port was cleaned thoroughly with the cleaning solution.

The following medicine, Adriamycin/Doxorubicin, is also known as the "Red Devil." This was the medicine that made you sick and caused you to lose all of your hair over time. I took a very heavy dosage of this chemical. Each treatment required that I take two syringes, each approximately one inch in diameter and a little over 6 inches in length. This chemical was the hardest to take out of all the medicines. The nurse would sit next to me and slowly administer this medicine one syringe at a time. It would take about 15-20 minutes to get through one tube. The nurse warned me about this chemical. She said that it would most likely cause me to feel nauseated and that when I went to urinate, my urine would be red. The nausea I had heard about, but the red urine I was not prepared for. When the nurse started to dispense the Red Devil, I could feel the chemical exit the port and enter the vein it was attached to. The chemical felt like warm syrup that I could feel traveling over every centimeter of my shoulder, under my arm, and into my heart. Then as the chemical entered the heart, it felt like my heart filled up like a water balloon. The feeling made my heart rate increase, and soon it felt like my heart was full of this warm syrup and immediately started pumping it out in what felt like several veins at the very same time. It felt like the warm thick chemical was being pushed out slowly into every vein and that I could track its movement in every vein that led to my stomach, each leg, and each arm. Once the chemical got to my stomach, I began to feeling a little nauseated. The nausea would stay with me 24 hours a day for the next six months' worth of treatments. After I made it through the first syringe, it was time for the second. After the completion of the second syringe, the port was cleaned with the solution.

Following the extended period of receiving the Red Devil, the nurse then hooked up an IV bag of the next chemical. This chemical was administered as a slow drip that could take a couple of hours. I learned through the process that if you sped up the drip from the IV bag, it would cause you to get a headache and increase your nausea significantly. I only tried this once as I thought I could take it, but once my head started hurting, and I felt as if the room was spinning, and my nausea increased, I asked if they could slow it back down because it was too much.

Usually, I had to use the restroom after the IV bag had started. I would have to get up and unplug the machine that monitored the IV bag. I would then roll the IV bag, hanging on this mobile metal coat hanger, around the corner to the bathroom. During these moments, the most disturbing events would repeatedly occur as long as I was taking the Red Devil. When you start to urinate, your urine stream is a deep red color. Although I was warned that the red urine would appear, there is nothing that really can prepare you on actually seeing it. I instantly thought there could be an issue with this. It shocked me because of the deep color of red. After I finished, I thoroughly washed my hands like I was a doctor preparing for surgery. When I returned to my chair, I told my mother about my red urine experience. I explained how creepy it was and that I was not looking forward to that experience while taking the chemotherapy treatments.

At the end of a chemical therapy session, the doctors would have had enough time to thoroughly analyze your blood results and would prescribe more medicine as needed. In one example, I had a session where my iron levels were low, and the doctor prescribed an IV bag of iron for me to take at the end of my chemical therapy session. This IV bag tacked on an additional hour to the average six and a half hours that I spent getting treatment already. Obviously, this was one of the days that I did not go back to work but instead went home to lie down after a long treatment session.

My second chemotherapy treatment was held at Clearview Cancer Institute (CCI). My oncologist split his time between Crestwood and the CCI. The experience was amazing. I remember pulling up to the facility and noticing how clean and modern the building appeared. The front of the entire building looked to be made of glass windows. There was a large water fountain in the center of what looked like a manmade mini pond. The landscape design appeared to be done by a top designer. There was a brick walkway surrounding the water, which seemed to make a smooth transition into the round-about pavement that circled in front of the main entrance. There was a large overhang that extended the full length of the building, which made it seem like I was pulling up to an airport to unload for a flight.

When you walked through the huge sliding double doors, there was a security guard right at the door next to a band of wheelchairs. He wore the typical earth toned uniform that was accompanied by a smile. The front entranceway of CCI was long enough where there was about six to eight doors with a waiting area in-between each door. Each waiting area was wide enough for a couch and two chairs on either side. As you walked in, you faced the check-in counter, where the ladies would always smile to display their pearly white teeth when they greeted you. As they would ask the typical name, date-of-birth questions, you could hear the compassion and concern levels in their voice. Every single visit was the exact same. I started to think that the only way someone could be employed at CCI was if they had passed an extended smile and courtesy test. Before long, they started to recognize me and greeted me by my name. The only thing I would have to answer at that point was my date-of-birth. Even the people who took the blood samples wore the same smile.

Every time I went, there would be all kinds of conversations going on. For example, it was basketball season, and we would briefly discuss college and professional basketball. We would make our personal Final Four and playoff predictions. One time, I met a former high school classmate in there that remembered me, but I could not remember her. There was another time that I went in to get my treatment's preliminary blood work, and the mood was a little somber between the technicians. I overheard them speaking about a patient that was in the hospital, and the doctors had determined hospice should be called in. The technicians who took the blood samples were talking about who all would be going to see the patient. It was so amazing to see how people who worked at CCI had a great level of concern for individuals who had been coming in there for extended periods of time. These people seemed to have a bond created with all the patients. By the time I would reach my final treatment, I told them I made it through, and they were glad that I made it through but surprised that the time seemed to pass quickly. It felt good that I was able to create what seemed like new found friends with the people who I only would spend about five minutes with during each of my CCI visits.

During my time at CCI, after completing my blood work, I typically would go cattycorner from the blood work area to register to see the doctor and make any necessary co-payments. I would then wait at Dr. Dang's patient area. The nurse that would be taking my vitals would come out of the magnetically secured door and call my name. They would then proceed to tell me to step on the digital scale to get my weight measurements. If I did not like the numbers, I would jokingly ask them if the scale had been calibrated recently. If they said that the machine had not been calibrated, I would say that it was overdue. If they said that the machine had been calibrated, I would say it was not calibrated correctly. We always got a little tickle from my jokes.

After taking the vitals, they would lead me to another section of the building where the chemotherapy treatments would be administered. I followed them down another hall where we walked between two glass pods (rooms) where all the nurses' stations were. This was where they kept track of patients' schedules and medicine orders. Once we cleared the glass pods, we stepped into the tiled aisle that led to different treatment pods. Each pod had approximately eight reclining leather chairs. The far wall was made of glass with a door that led to the rear of the building. The rear of the building had what looked like a grassy park with a concrete brook on the far side of the walkway. It was an inspirational scene in the springtime.

Like at Crestwood, I was able to pick any chair to sit in for my chemotherapy treatment. I would always first look to see if any chairs next to the glass paned wall were open. I loved nature. As you chose your location for treatment, you would sit and repeat your treatment's routine. All of my remaining treatments were held at the CCI because of my experience during my second chemotherapy treatment.

So many inspirational events occurred at CCI. Volunteers could always been seen pushing carts full of snacks and juices. The carts also had heated compartments that would carry blankets for the patients receiving treatments. I met a lady who had breast cancer over 30 years prior to us meeting and never had a chemotherapy or radiation treatment. She only had a surgery to remove the tumor. As I got to know her, my community outreach led our conversations into topics about providing opportunities to underserviced areas in the city. Since then, we developed a valuable outreach partnership that is still active to this day.

Sometimes while at CCI for treatments, I would see people come for treatment without a partner, friend, or family member. Too often, it would be an elderly individual. The good thing about the volunteers is that they would talk to you about anything just to accompany the person who was going through the treatment. I remember seeing an elderly man who was dropped off by a cab and would be taking treatments for most of the day. I saw an elderly couple that would come in together. The husband would be taking treatments for more than 8 hours in a day. I would return to CCI the next morning to get a steroid shot, and I would see the same elderly couple that had returned the very next day to take more hours of treatments. I would later find out that he was in the advanced stages of cancer. There were teenage girls who looked like the cheerleader type and some who looked like they had received a multitude of scholarships for their academic achievements. This disease did not discriminate.

On one occasion, I had a very rough treatment session. I was leaning forward in the reclining chair, slowly rocking back and forth, almost in the fetal position. I was sick to my stomach. My eyes were closed. I happened to open my eyes, and I saw a young little boy who could not have been older than eight years old. He was walking to the bathroom playing a handheld game while his dad was pushing the mobile IV cart behind him. Instantly, I was shocked to see such a young boy in CCI taking treatments. I began to think, *If this young boy can do what is necessary and take this, I know I can*. I knew he was experiencing a level of discomfort similar to me, yet here he was walking and playing the game like there was nothing going on. His pace was solid, his focus was on the game, and he looked as if he did not have a care in the world. At that moment, my faith kicked in to remind me that I had been chosen to walk this path. So, no matter the discomfort I had to endure, it was expected. I was inspired by the young boy playing a video game; he had a positive effect on my mentality to fight this cancer. I knew I had to be continually strong in order to make it. My faith spawned my belief that the victory was already mine. I only had to proceed through the expected difficult process.

Going through so many hours of chemical therapy treatment meant that there were many hours/days of work that were going to be missed. Because it was the start of a new year, I didn't have any vacation or sick leave hours to use. This meant I had to figure out how I would do my treatments, work, and have the funds to pay for all the unexpected expenses that could, and would, occur. When I started my treatments, I thought that if I could receive treatments and finish before 2:30 p.m., then I could get to work by 3 and work 3 to 4 hours before going home. I knew my miscellaneous savings account would come in handy. I didn't expect, however, that I would eventually have to pull from my emergency savings account as well. My mentality was to do whatever I had to do to get through this trial. In hindsight, I realized that I was not always thinking clearly. However, I was trying to figure out the best decisions in a short time. I did check on getting short-term disability while going through treatments, but I found out that I had to be out of work for four to six months before payments would start being issued. That was not acceptable at the time because I could keep working and still receive more support from a short payment cycle than the payments from the short-term disability. This was what initiated my drive to continue to work while going through therapy treatments.

I was blessed to have people who helped me along this journey. When I learned that I had cancer and would have to go through therapy treatments, I told Mr. Lloyd Brooks first, and he gave me a lot of useful information. Then later, while walking down to another building on our campus, I saw my manager. After getting his attention, I told him about my cancer diagnosis and that I needed to go through chemotherapy. I could see him, as he was processing the news, tearing up but trying to remain strong. He said he was so sorry to hear the news. But I continued to wear a smile for the both of us. I told him everything would be all right, and I would keep him posted.

A few weeks after telling my manager about the news, I was sitting at my desk when an email popped up on my computer screen from my manager. It stated that he had reached out to the company's leadership, and my situation was communicated across the entire company (in multiple sites all over the United States). People all over the company donated over 100 hours of leave for me to use while I went through treatment. When I read this, my mouth dropped. I immediately teared up because I could not believe that so many people whom I had never met would be willing to give me hours to help me go through this trial. I immediately wrote a response for him to send out across the company that would express my thanks to everyone. I had to wish everyone God's Blessings. What a very unexpected, pleasant surprise. This was another testimony of evidence that serving a giving God pays off. He will never put more on you than you can bear. He knows the needs of his children and will provide. It may not be in our time, but it is always *on time*.

CHAPTER 5 | THE EFFECTS OF CHEMOTHERAPY

Chemical therapy can take a heavy toll on the body, and it can affect everyone in different ways and to different extents. For one, chemical therapy brings the immune system down. It does not take long before you start feeling the effects of the therapy. It brings down your immune system in a way I like to call the roller coaster affect. If you are familiar with a roller coaster, you know that the highest point of a roller coaster is at the beginning. The ride is full of bends, turns, loops, and different speeds, but it never reaches the same height as it started. Well, your immune system endures the same concept. At the beginning of your chemical therapy series, your immune system is at peak performance. As you begin your journey, the first session brings down your immune system. After the session, the immune system is trying get back to the level as it was before but does not quite make it before the next session. Each session is another hill encountered that is not as quite as tall as the previous hill you were on. In comparison, your immune system never reaches the performance level that it achieved the session before. Due to a lower immune system, you have to be increasingly careful with the number of people you come in contact with. You also have to be very careful of receiving germs. That is why you are instructed to have a lot of Germ-X to keep your hands a clean as possible. They also tell you to avoid big crowds. Buffet style eating is frowned upon because of the increased chance of getting germs. With a consistently lowering immune system, you are capable of becoming sick very easily.

During the very first treatment, I began feeling a little funny, but by the end of the treatment, I felt like I was fighting an illness and had to regurgitate everything in my stomach. Imagine feeling nausea 24 hours a day, 7 days a week for 6 months. Once that feeling started, it never left until approximately two weeks after my last treatment. When you wake up in the morning to the time you lie down and finally go to sleep, you feel like you don't want to make any swift movements or lie down in the wrong way as if one wrong move would make you sick. I was very conscious and careful of the food I consumed because it could possibly make me sick, too.

During my chemotherapy treatments, I remember having a heightened sense of smell. People say that when one of the human senses is weakened, another sense tends to get stronger. My sense of smell increased to the level that whenever I smelled certain things from extraordinary distances, my nausea would become harder to contain. It was hard for me to be around people who wore cologne or perfume. I tried to fight through the discomfort of smells around me, but too often, I would I have to leave the area I was in. Sometimes, I would have to remind my mother that she was wearing too much perfume, but it was not her amount she put on but my extreme level of smell that was heightened. My nose would burn, causing me to sneeze and itch. There were times that my mother would be cooking in my home, and

I could not be in or near the kitchen while she was cooking. The smell would be too overbearing. I would have to be in my room about 60 feet away.

Other times, while going to CCI or Crestwood for treatments or follow-ups, I could smell the chemicals used for therapy in the parking lot. Usually, the smell would hit me as soon as I got out of the car. This was one of the craziest feelings that I had experienced during the chemical treatments. I would be outside, hundreds of feet away from where the chemicals would be administered on the inside of the building. Imagine that you get out of your car and into the open air, and you can smell the chemicals that are approximately a 40-yard walk to the front door, through another door 20 yards within the building, down a 20-yard hallway, and to another section of the building where they house the chemicals for therapy. I began to think that I and a shark shared one significant ability: to smell blood in the ocean miles away.

I believe my heightened sense of smell was manifested from the degradation of my sense of feel. Neuropathy in my hands and feet started to set in after my twelfth chemical therapy session. I had 16 sessions scheduled. I remember having the option of doing 12 or 16 sessions. They say hindsight is 20/20. I look back on things now, and I wish I had chosen the 12 sessions because now I still have everlasting effects like neuropathy from doing all 16 sessions. I remember in the week that followed my twelfth chemical therapy session, my hands started to feel funny, as if they were asleep from me laying on them. The only difference was that I could not shake them hard enough to get the blood flowing and awaken the nerves in my hands. After the thirteenth session, my feet started to feel the same way. I lost feeling in my feet. Not having feeling in your hands and feet is a dangerous situation to be in. I remember looking at my hand one day as I was home, taking my finger and slowly bending it backwards to see if it would start hurting, and I had no sensation whatsoever. My hands had lost all of their feelings. Imagine holding a cup and having it fall from your grasp because you are not sure how much pressure you are putting to the cup. I had a drink fall from my grasp a few times. For this reason, I had to make sure to focus on what I was doing and sometimes use my other hand to put under the bottom of the cup to ensure that I did not drop it.

Neuropathy was the same for my feet and toes. This is so dangerous because you can step on something, and the wound can get infected if you are not checking your feet. For this reason, I had to watch everywhere I stepped, and additionally, I had to make sure that I never dropped anything around the house. I was constantly vacuuming the house. I always checked my socks and shoes before putting them on, and I made sure to wear something on my feet if I ever walked anywhere in or out of the house.

The chemical therapy also made me lose the nails on my feet and hands. This effect manifested within the first month of treatments. My nails started turning a yellowish tinted color first then a dark tinted hue of a couple of weeks after. Before long, the nails became really brittle and would easily crack or become disengaged with my finger. There were some spots under the finger and toenails that were still engaged with the skin and would start bleeding if you pulled or tugged at the nail. Fortunately, this side effect occurred before the neuropathy set in. Pulling at your finger and toenails without having feeling would have caused more damage than when you do having feeling in your extremities. Eventually, my nails would grow back in lieu of the chemical therapy. In some cases, my toenails grew back in an awkward manner but would straighten out within a few months.

Along with the loss of my nails, my skin became chalky, dark, and easy to crack in many areas. It was hard to moisturize. The lotion that I was using was working well enough. I remember having a conversation with one of my community outreach colleagues who I was in graduate school with, and she talked to me about some better lotion to use. She actually turned me on to using Nivea lotion products. I started using the more therapeutic lotion that significantly helped me stay moisturized.

Unfortunately, the therapeutic lotion could not help my skin from becoming a shade darker, especially around my knuckles and eyes. It took a few months after my last chemical therapy session for my skin tone and nails to return to somewhat normal. Years later, I still have issues with one toenail growing back normal, and I still have dark spots around my eyes. I have just accepted that this is something I will have to deal with.

Something that was easier to deal with for me personally was the loss of all of my hair. I had been shaving my head with a razor since high school. I occasionally would wear a mustache or a little chin hair but rarely a full beard. So, I was accustomed to not having a lot of facial hair. I was not accustomed to having every single hair removed across my entire body. That includes eyebrows, eyelashes, nose hair, arm pits, and private areas. The strangest thing about the loss of hair is that it will catch you off guard when it starts coming out. I had very thick and bushy eyebrows with a slight hint of a unibrow. I remember one day waking up to wash my face and looking in the towel and having hair all over it like I had just got done shaving. I stared at the towel for what felt like 10 minutes. I remember running my thumb across the towel as if the hairs were not real, and I needed verification. I immediately looked in the mirror at my face and could instantly tell the density of my eyebrows had become thinner. My first feeling was of despair and hurt. I became a little down. I remember walking back to my bed and looking at my pillow to find more hairs on the pillowcase and sheets. This moment can be a little disheartening when you normally do not find any hairs on the pillowcases. I was fortunate enough to be in a relationship with someone who would help bring a different perspective to a lot of situations, not barring the hair loss.

When I first told her that my hair was coming out, she said to me, "You expected that, right? Well don't worry about it. It will be easier for you to manscape (Google it) now, Brazilian style."

I could not do anything but laugh at her welcomed inappropriate joke. Who in the world would say that? She knew how to lighten my mood and make me feel better.

Potatoes and milkshakes also made me feel better during my chemical therapy sessions. One of the side effects of taking the chemical therapy sessions was that I lost taste for a majority of foods. The only things that had a taste to me were potatoes and milkshakes.

I really believed that having a positive attitude and an uplifted spirit would help me beat this disease. Anytime I could find happiness, I made sure to pursue it during the difficult times. If I could have potatoes during this journey, I would make sure to eat them. I remember while going through some chemical therapy sessions, I'd ask my best friend and brother from another mother BJ to bring my Chick-fil-A waffle fries. This guy never failed me during my hard times. I love those waffle fries, about as much as I love my brother. Usually, when I got home after a chemical therapy session, I would eat my mother's homemade potato soup. She would also make enough for me to take to work.

I also ate baked potatoes and potato casseroles. In addition to the potatoes, I loved homemade milkshakes. This was something that I usually would not drink in large quantities, but when you are going through something heavy, I found this was the one sugar-filled treat that I could actually taste and was truly comforting. I probably had a homemade milkshake once a day. I believe this was a huge mistake as the chemical therapy reduced the performance of all my organs, specifically my pancreas. It is suspected that I all of my glucose consumption could have induced a fight with diabetes. I previously was not a diabetic. My type 2 diabetic adventure did not start until after my string of chemical therapy treatments. I partially blame the fact that I did not fully understand the situation, which I was not as prepared for as I would have liked. During the treatment, I was looking for any pleasure to help my constant mental battles.

No matter how strong I would be one minute, negative thoughts would consistently creep into my mind. I constantly pondered if people's actions were directly related to their perception of my situation. It is my opinion that people of the world often shy away from sickness and disease, mainly due to the lack of knowledge and/or understanding, and it creates a subliminal fear within the individual. This is where the strength of the fearful individual's mentality will allow them to move into feared situations. Those who have knowledge and understanding of some situations ideally do not carry the same level of fear. In my case, I lacked a full understanding of how cancer is birthed, exists, and the ways to impede its mutation. The fear of not knowing what to expect was present in my mind most hours in the day. At times, it was hard to focus or to find true happiness throughout the day, so I eagerly welcomed any moment of happiness that appeared.

During my chemical therapy treatments, I would welcome talking and seeing the special lady in my life at the time. She was my breath of fresh air. She was very comforting and supportive in ways that I could not get from family or my caregiver. It appeared that our energy connection was strengthened. Our emotional bond seemed to be more in tune. Cancer will make you appreciate the little things like the time spent with a person. You cherish every single second. Needless to say that during these times of heightened emotional connections, the sexual encounters are extremely intense. Love is expressed in a way beyond anything routine. Each time feels like that is the last time you have to say, "I love you." Time is not taken for granted; therefore, you make the most of every minute. Every love expression episode was so emotionally and physically draining. I remember being so exhausted at times because chemical therapy sessions would drain my energy levels. Even immediately following a chemical therapy session, we would find time to express our love for one another. As the treatments approached an end, the harder it was to recover in energy for the following week.

I remember that it was increasingly harder to get through the days due to my energy level never returning to par from the previous day. Imagine being a cell phone and you have a predetermined energy level to expend on whatever tasks that had to be done. Once expended, you are done until you recharge. There is no go to overdrive or start tapping into the reserve. There is no reserve. Toward the end of my sessions my cousin was getting married five hours away from where I stayed. I always told him whenever he got married I would be there. I had a therapy session that lasted most of the day on Thursday. My mother drove me down the following day, and I was exhausted, but I had a wedding to be in. I went to rehearsal that Friday night. The rehearsal was not that bad as I was able to keep sitting down between my escorting the bridesmaid. I attempted to go to the bachelor party, but I did not make it all the way through. I had to stand the entire time I was there, and about 50 guys in a small area surrounded me. I already was not supposed to be around large crowds because of my chemotherapy. I proceeded to find my cousin to tell him I was going back to my room so I could lie down. He understood and was grateful I attempted to hang out with him. I told him if the entertainment had not showed up late I might have made it. Seriously, I would have walked out in the middle of the show because I was just barely standing after the long day. The following day, I made it through the wedding, but I was barely holding on. Between standing for the party's entrance and the wedding itself, I felt like I had to battle my legs for energy just standing there.

By the time we left for the reception, I was just happy to sit in the car to go to the reception. The time to rest felt very good on my aching legs. When we arrived at the reception hall, we had to stand in the main lobby for an extended period of time before the reception. Although every minute of standing was extremely draining, it was a little entertaining to see some of the bridesmaids criticizing the wedding coordinator who eventually started responding to the criticism. Tempers started to rise to an extreme high just before it was time to go in. Miraculously, they were able to put their difference of opinions aside so the wedding party could walk in. Regardless, I made it through the event and was so glad to get back to the hotel to sleep like a baby. I was still living my life as best as I could, but I was in no way expecting or prepared for what was about to come around the corner.

CHAPTER 6 | THE ACCIDENT

In preparation for my treatments, I wanted to get my mental and physical together for the long battle. I decided to start seeing a chiropractor once I began chemical therapy so I could get my central nervous system in line and in the best performance grade possible. The previous winter, I took in an informative seminar on the importance of having spinal therapy and the benefits of consistently treating the spinal cord. The chiropractor that I chose made every visit a very enjoyable experience. The spinal doctor that I used for my spinal treatments believes in natural healing. He does not use manufactured medicine for his entire family. The human body is an amazing, self-healing organism. Therefore, it needs to be in the best operating status possible to help fight injury and disease.

I do believe that seeing the chiropractor served many benefits while I was going through my chemical therapy. After learning the condition of my spine and treating it properly, I was able to determine how I could relieve tension in certain locations while sleeping. This allowed me to get much better sleep at night so I could feel as refreshed as possible during my challenging times. Although I was working my way through the chemical therapy by being proactive in my diet and body, I also tried to satisfy my mental stability by maintaining my community involvement with engineering societies, professional organizations, and the local school board's advisory committee. I also wanted to make sure I maintained my level of enjoyable hobbies like motorcycling. Unfortunately, the thing that brought me great pleasure was about to bring me great pain.

In May, I was past the midway point of my chemical therapy. It was a beautiful day with pretty nice weather, and I had been invited to the graduation party of my church member's eldest son. I had been playing basketball with this church member for years. We played together in several locations. It was a Sunday, and I remember debating if I was going to ride my motorcycle or drive the car. Since I just had the bike custom painted and the helmets to match, I thought the high school kids would like to see the bike. As I contemplated whether to ride the bike, I was unsure if I was going to wear all of my protective gear. I decided not to bring all the protective gear to help keep me from wanting to do bike tricks at the party. In the end, I left with just a helmet, some jeans, and a baseball jersey.

I called Jordan to see what time his party was going to start. I could hear his mother in the background saying, "Tell him that it starts right now." I told him I was on my way and that I would be riding the bike. After hanging up with him, I called my mother and asked where she was and if she was going to the party. She said she was on her way. I told her I was getting ready to leave, and I would meet her over there.

As I rode in heavy traffic on a two-lane road, I became aware of a car that was tailgating me. I repeatedly looked behind me to see how close the car was. I decided to move up to give us some separation. I wanted to make sure we had a few car lengths between us. When I looked back, I heard tires screeching on the pavement, so I immediately turned around to see what was going on. I saw the van in front of me doing a nosedive like it was about to have an accident. In an unreal instant, calculations were made in a second. I remember thinking I could move to the left, but I could not see if traffic was coming. I could move to the right and go into the ditch, but there was a metal grate somewhere coming, and I could not tell how far it was. I would have to use the front brake, which would induce a "Stoppie" maneuver, but I didn't believe I had enough clearance to bring it down without taking a header into the van.

In the next second, I decided to try to go for the front brake to stop, but I did not have the clearance. In a split second, I realized I was stopping with my back wheel in the air, and I had a decision to make: either keep trying to stop or release the brake and hit the back of the vehicle. I decided to try and stop, but I was still coming up too fast, so I decided to go over the top of the motorcycle. As I went over the top of my motorcycle, I tucked and rolled over my left shoulder. It seemed like everything was moving in slow motion. As I hit the pavement, I started to roll from shoulder to shoulder, and as I got to my second roll I remember thinking, *That bike is coming,* and as soon as the thought came to my mind, I felt the bike hit my back and slide down my lower back and hit my leg. Right after I tumbled one more time, I could see the bike sliding below me toward the van. Then I slid to a stop while laying on my left shoulder as if I was sleeping on my side. I immediately tried to keep from blacking out by shaking my head and fighting to keep my eyes open. After I got my bearings from what seemed like the world was spinning, I tried to get up, but I could not. I paused for a brief second then tried to get up again, but I could not. Immediately, I thought something was wrong. I wiggled the toes in my left foot to see my boot move. I then wiggled the toes in my right foot to see my boot move. I tried to get up again, and I could not. I grew increasingly nervous.

While trying to pull my helmet off, I saw a lady running toward me. She was yelled, "Don't move." She asked me was I ok when she got up to me. I told her I thought I might be ok, but I could not move my right leg. I did not want to move my left leg because my right leg was lying on top of it. She said that they were calling the ambulance, and it was on the way. It turned out she was a nurse that worked at the nursing home up the road and came down when she saw the accident. I remember reaching in my right pocket to get out my phone so I could call and tell my mother what happened. I thought if she could hear from me rather than a stranger then she would not be hysterical about the news. As I called her, using what I did not realize was the hand on my broken forearm, the lady took the phone to tell her what happened. While she was on the phone, a black off duty cop ran up while a black female helped redirect traffic. After she got off the phone, she said, "I let your mother know what's happened, and she's going to meet you at the hospital." She smiled reassuringly and added, "You are doing so well. Continue to keep calm."

When the EMS got there, they asked what happened, and some lady replied that someone had walked into the street, and the cars were stopping to keep from hitting the man. The EMS personnel immediately cut my pants leg open and said that my leg was definitely broken. They were going to have to put me on the transport board. After they strapped me on the board and from the waist up. They said they were getting ready to pick me up, and I told them, "Please make sure you hold my leg when you pick me up." The strap was across my thigh, just above the break.

I heard someone say they got it before they counted, "One... two... three... lift."

As they picked me up, my right leg flopped to the right side of my body, above the knee where the break was. It was hanging to the side as if I was sitting up on the edge of a bed. The EMS guy tried to quickly push it back, but I was already yelling by that time. This was the worst pain I had ever felt in my life. I was not in pain until that moment. My femur was broken in half. My leg looked like something out of a cartoon. It was unreal.

By the time I got to the emergency room, the EMS team told me what was going to happen next and would not leave until they talked to the doctor. It was not long before they cut all my clothes off. When the doctor arrived, he stated that there would be some interns coming in. As I was laying on a freezing cold table inside a room that felt like a meat locker, I remember looking toward the door, and it seemed like there were nothing but young ladies examining my leg. I was more concerned to let them know I normally carry more length in my manhood. The pain was too great for me to say anything. After the doctor's inspection, he informed me that I broke my right forearm, right femur, and my left shoulder. Come to find out that the chemical therapy made my bones brittle and easy to break. Months later, I would find out that I also cracked my hip.

Before too long, they let my mother, my other brother from another mother Vense, BJ, and my dad back in the emergency area. I did not see all the people who came to the emergency room, but my friends said it was about 100 people there. It was good to feel that much love from the community. My family had yet to be notified other than my mother and dad. A lot of these people were friends in the community and people I met while motorcycling over the years. There were more representatives from each motorcycle group that showed up than the group that I used to be the vice president of. Of those former members of that particular group, I established true friendship with those individuals. The confirmed lesson here is that people will say anything, but people who truly care about you will show up without asking. I had no clue then how so many people knew I had the accident nor did I know so many people I barely knew cared that much. They stayed with my mother for hours and were in and out of the emergency room. People from all my walks of life showed up at the hospital.

It was decided that my surgeries would occur the next day because the preferred surgeon would be in that Monday. That night in my room was a difficult one. Several people came to the room, and it was hard to maneuver. Whenever I tried to move my broken leg in the bed, it felt like a wiggling nub within my thigh that was extremely painful. When I had to adjust my position in the bed, I had to use the overhead assist bar. Unfortunately, my left shoulder was broke, and I could not put my left arm over my head, so I had to use my right arm with the broken forearm to pull myself up. Interestingly enough, I was blessed not to feel any pain in my forearm. They told me I should not be using it, but I had no other choice to move around in the bed. Sleeping was more difficult. Whenever I would lean to my left, my shoulder would swell up like the Hunchback of Notre Dame. I would have to move over to the right side to let the swelling go down. I was doing this back and forth movement all night.

While in the hospital, my oncologist came to visit me before my next treatment. He informed me that due to my accident and upcoming surgeries, there was no need to do the chemical therapy that week, but we would resume the same time the following week. I asked the oncologist that since my bones were broken, if there was a possibility of the cancer spreading to my bones. He ensured me that the cancer would not spread to my bones. I felt slightly relieved, but I still had a little suspicion that it could be possible. That was just another moment that doubt was setting in.

After my surgeries, I had to get accustomed to my recovery lifestyle. I had a plate placed in my right forearm and a brace applied on the outside. I was not supposed to lift anything heavy with that arm. My right leg had a titanium rod put through my femur, which was inserted through the hip. Two screws held the rod in place just above the knee and one screw close to the hip. You could see the obvious break of the femur on the X-ray and the two pieces separated by approximately a half an inch. I was instructed not to put any pressure on my leg for several weeks. So I was given a walker with a cradle for my right arm. The interesting thing about the walker was that it required me to hold myself up with my left side—the side with a broken shoulder that was yet to be operated on because the operating doctor didn't think it was broke. So for two weeks, I continued to go to my chemical therapy treatments with a damaged shoulder. The nurses and technicians at CCI asked me what happened when they saw me limping in with my walker. When I explained that I had a motorcycle accident, they asked me if I quit riding. The answer was a simple no. I often responded, "If you get bucked by a horse, you don't get rid of the horse—you keep riding."

I finally went to my orthopedic doctor and told him about my shoulder. After he looked at my X-rays, he quickly determined my shoulder was broke, and I had to have surgery as soon as possible. The surgery provided a tremendous relief of pain to my shoulder, and I could go through the treatments somewhat easier.

It was just as difficult to go to the chiropractor. I could not lie on the table on my left shoulder, so we had to work around that minor issue. The funny thing about the accident is that the chiropractor noticed something very strange from the X-rays they took immediately following the accident. He noted that my spine was more inline since the accident than it was before the accident. He could not believe what he was looking at and pulled up both films so I could see. I could also see the noticeable difference between the two films. From that point on, he started calling me Superman. He was very shocked at the progress I was making through it all. The chiropractic treatments were a huge tension release each time I went. I could definitely feel a positive effect from the weekly treatments. Each time I would go, the chiropractor would ask me about the chemical therapy treatments and how my body was reacting to the medicine. I informed him that even though I was nauseated all the time, I could tell that my nausea would decrease significantly within 24 hours after getting a spinal adjustment. Although I was getting more in debt by continuing my treatments, I chose to keep them going until the end of my chemical therapy treatments.

The bills definitely started piling up during the chemical therapy treatments. I had to pay for the all the medicine I took for multiple side effects. I had to pay copays each time I went to my oncologist, my orthopedic doctor, or the emergency surgeon. I had to pay for each chiropractor visit. I had to pay for my hospital deductibles, all blood work done at CCI, and I also had to maintain my own household bills while making sure my daughter's child support was paid. Having cancer exponentially multiplies pressure and added stress to a person's life. The financial burden can weight just as heavily on you as the frightening thoughts of chemotherapy, radiation, death, and leaving those you love behind. This is where things can be increasingly hard to handle mentally. There were several months where the bills became too much to bear, and the savings account became drained extremely fast. There were points where I had to ask for a little help. I hated to have to ask for help, and I definitely didn't (and still don't) like owing anyone anything. I made sure that when I got back on my feet I would pay back all my debts. Those financial gifts that the givers would not allow me to pay back to them, I paid it forward in various ways. The main thing about the financial burden of going through cancer is that there is funding out there to help you. You just have to do the research to find it. Ask as many questions as you can. Just do your part and have the faith—God will deliver right on time— in many areas beyond financial.

The end of my chemical therapy treatments came during the Fourth of July weekend. Although I had been dealing with the neuropathy in my hands and feet, I was still feeling good that I had made it to the end of the treatments. It was perfect when I leaned that one of my childhood friends and his brother came home to his Samoan parents' house, and my mother and I were invited to their house to celebrate the Fourth. For this, this was a time to celebrate the end of my treatments, the Fourth, and the reconnecting with friends. So, we went to visit them, and a lot of my old childhood friends were there. We had a great time. It was the first time a lot of them had seen me since I found out that I had cancer and also had the bike accident. We had a great time reconnecting. I remember thinking that there are always those friends whom you can count on when the chips are down. There were so many *so-called* friends who stopped coming around when I got sick. By the time my mother and I left the get-together, I confirmed, yet again, who really mattered in my life.

My mother drove us to my place as I was loaded up on medicine. As we got close to my house, my phone started ringing. It was the team captain on the flag football team, the Blackhawks—the team I played on when I found the knot in my chest. I only knew Ryan from the gym, so I was wondering why he was calling me. As I picked up the phone, we started conversing about the gym and how the guys at the gym found out that I had cancer and a motorcycle accident. Ryan proceeded to tell me that they guys were pulling for me, and if I needed anything (e.g., my grass cut, cars washed, errands to run), to let them know, and they would do it. I was shocked by the offer, but what followed next shocked me even more.

I replied to the gracious offer: "Thank you. If I need something, I will definitely call you."

"Hey, what are you doing today?" Ryan asked.

I told him that I was just leaving one of my friend's BBQ and heading home.

"Well, that's good," he replied. "I was just making sure you were not alone for the Fourth. If you were, I was going to offer that I come and pick you up so you can spend the Fourth with me and my family."

My mouth dropped a little. I was stunned. I could not believe he said that. I tried to respond and tell him that it was much appreciated, but I don't believe I got all the words out smoothly without my voice cracking a little. I was getting choked up because someone I hardly knew was extending his family time to me so I would not be alone. This came at a time when I was easily angered to watch a number of people stop coming around and stop returning my calls. I never called for anything other than conversation and now that was too much to ask for. Now given you never know what someone is going through, I pray that it was for a decent reason other than what was more evident. God put Ryan in the perfect place at the perfect time to make me remember that I cannot get down when people are not in the places we would want them, but he will put them the right person in the right place at the right time.

It took my mother to tell me that I should not give up on people so quickly. Although I might have been going through "Chemo Brain" at the time, which raised my aggression level back to an all-time high, I still had to consider what the other side looked like. By definition from the Mayo Clinic, Chemo Brain is a cognitive impairment or cognitive dysfunction that is chemical therapy related; it induces thinking and memory problems while raising aggression levels. I would find myself snapping at my mother who was a caregiver and sometimes at my lady. I would have to come back and apologize to both of them often after I thought of my actions. However, I did not view it that way with a lot of my friends not being there as I would hope they would.

First, my mother had to make me realize that a lot of my friends were used to seeing me active, strong, and independent. To see me now sick, extremely weak, and dependent on others was scary for them. The human nature of fear is a powerful feeling that can subliminally take control over anyone. It is the expression of fear that may differ from person to person. My mother explained to me that a lot of people really do not know what to say or do when they see someone down and hurting. Several people will shy away from sickness, especially a *big* sickness like cancer because it is often a disease that is not understood. This reminded me of a quote from an unknown source I repeated for years: "Fear is the lack of knowledge." It is based on the premise that it is the items of the world that you don't understand that often brings fear. However, Leo Tolstoy may be more correct in saying "Do not fear the lack of knowledge, but rear false knowledge." Regardless, I initially found myself disappointed and hurt that the individuals I would rather be there were not there when I could have used them the most.

Second, I was reminded again on looking at things in another perspective. Although some of my friends might have been given the gift of fear, there were others that just would not be there because of who they were, even though I wanted them there. After my chemical therapy treatments were complete, I remember meeting an elderly man whom I had a long conversation with. As we talked and I shared my story of having breast cancer as a male, finishing chemical therapy, and losing out on a lot of so-called friends, I realized I was stronger and better mentally now. I had a way to go in my physical recovery, but I was going to be so much better due to people shunning me. I was having a beat-on-your-chest (Tarzan) moment. I am sure the elder gentleman could hear it in the tone of my voice.

As I talked, the older man did not say anything; he just kept looking down at his Bible. When I completed my last sentence of how strong I was, while he was looking down, he said, "Have you ever had a puzzle?"

Perplexed by his question, I answered yes.

"Have you ever had one of those big puzzles that had more than 100 pieces?"

Still being perplexed by his question, I stated yes.

"You ever found a piece of the puzzle that looked like it fit in one spot and you try to push it down, but it does not go?"

I replied yes.

"So, you take your thumb and try to push down on it. You pick it up, examine it, rotate it, and try to push it back down with your thumb, but it just does not quite fit?"

I said yeah.

"Well, people are often times like pieces of a puzzle. We often try to put them in places in our lives we want them to fit, but they were not made to fit there. You cannot get mad at people for being who they are."

I instantly dropped my mouth. In those words, in that moment, I got it. Every single relationship in life could now be defined.

We cannot get mad at who people are. People come in so many different shapes, sizes, personalities, and carry many different levels of beliefs/standards. No matter how much we would like for a person to fit in a certain place in our life, they will fit where they are supposed to fit. We cannot force them to fit in a place that they do not belong. When the time is right, the right puzzle piece will be provided to slip right in. So, the popular saying holds true, "If it does not fit, don't force it." At this point, I had a more forgiving heart, and I could move on in life with a better understanding of handling person-to-person interactions.

CHAPTER 7 | GETTING BACK

Tamoxifen was the name of the drug that I had to take at the end of my chemical therapy treatments. I was supposed to take this drug for five years based on the studies that had been conducted. The unfortunate thing about a lot of those studies is that they are mainly, if not solely, conducted on an all-women segment. The two greatly interesting things about having to take Tamoxifen are that most insurance companies will not purchase the drug for a male and you will develop hot flashes. Insurance companies will not purchase Tamoxifen for males because it is identified as a drug solely for women. Therefore, men have to pay the full cost. The other interesting Tamoxifen fact is that it can cause you to have hot flashes. The financial burden of taking the drug can be overwhelming. However, the physical challenges of men battling hot flashes are very extreme, especially men with a shaved head.

The hot flashes were very extreme and lasted the full duration of taking Tamoxifen. I now know what women feel like who have to deal with hot flashes all the time. Hot flashes can come at any time during the day or night. You have to start preparing for those untimely hot flashes during any event that you may attend. I had to start carrying a handkerchief with me wherever I would go to wipe the sweat off of my baldhead. The thing about having a baldhead is there is no hair to catch the minor sweat beads; therefore, you appear to sweat far more than the next person. People would ask me if I was hot all the time. I would tell them it comes on quick because of the medicine I was taking–as to not be specific. I would be running organization meetings and have to remember my presentation training when sweating a lot. I often would use my Tamoxifen regiment as an icebreaker to let the audience know that I was sweating because of the medicine and not because I appeared to be nervous for being in front of a large audience.

To get back to my original life, I tried to resume my original capacity of community involvement. I continued to pursue my dream of having a fully funded summer engineering camp for kids. This is one of the goals that I used to help me get through the uphill battle of chemical therapy. I had started the effort of starting the camp the year before I found out that I had cancer. Although I encountered a breast cancer fight along the way, I would not give up in what I believed in. I was the president of the local chapter of the National Society of Black Engineers (NSBE) Professionals while I was going through my cancer fight. Between chemical therapy and the accident, I only missed one meeting during my two-year term. The most challenging experience while going through the cancer and being the leader of the professional chapter of NSBE would be standing through our scholarship banquet while in chemical therapy. Although the banquet would bring its own level of service satisfaction, the engineering camp was a larger than life project.

The initial efforts to get major corporations to back the camp resulted in verbal support but financially neglect. I would not let that stop me from continuing to pursue a way to have the camp. With the help of two engineers who shared my same vision, we were able to find resources to help us piece together our very first camp of seventy-seven kids that came from all over the northern part of the state. The weeklong camp was so successful that it captured the eyes of our local city school system. While meeting with the superintendent, serendipitously, we had the same vision for serving our community and growing the camp. With 100% financial support from our local school system, we grew the camp from seventy-seven kids in one location to six hundred kids in three locations all in one week. We have triangulated the entire city to afford all of kids the opportunity to attend the camp. Our next goal is to expand into the entire northern part of the state. The initiative will take some time to develop, which may go beyond my recovery to being back to full capabilities.

Chemical therapy can impede the body's healing as well as possibly hinder organs; this was a lesson learned while I was recovering from the surgeries performed due to the motorcycle accident. Apparently two major side effects that I encountered were that all of my bones were not healing at a normal rate, and I had developed type II diabetes. This became another contributor of why my femur had the hardest time healing. My femur seemed to not be healing across the gap, but we decided to give it more time to see if it would eventually catch up to the other bones' progress. All of my other bones seemed to heal as expected.

I did break a wire in my repaired shoulder as I was doing rehabilitation on my shoulder and leg that same year. Since I was due to have another shoulder surgery, I asked my orthopedic doctor would it be ok if we had the surgery to remove the port at the same time. He said he would contact the general surgeon that put the port in and see if they could coordinate a day.

I remember waking up after having the shoulder surgery and noticing my port was removed, but something was wrong. My shoulder felt much better, but I could not feel the right side of my face. I also could not swallow or speak properly. I was so frightened that I did not know what to think. After we conversed with the doctor, he believed I might have had some type of nerve damage in my neck because of the way they had my neck positioned and strapped down during surgery. I felt a little better that the doctor believed it would eventually get better, but he was not sure of the timeline. He did want to keep monitoring my progress. The anesthesiologist also was concerned about my condition and continued to check on me in the upcoming weeks. The numbness in the neck made it very hard to swallow any hard food. I was forced to having a soup diet for approximately five weeks. I gradually started getting feeling back in my face and neck. I was so ecstatic to be able to eat and speak again. Not being able to speak easily or being able to eat any kind of food brought an increased appreciation for having what functionality that I did have. There are so many people in the world who have so many other things going on at a much larger scale than I was dealing with. This event was another experience to why I didn't (and still don't) take the little things for granted and appreciate what I do have. Even with the challenges that *will* come up, things could always be worse.

As I restarted rehabilitation on my shoulder and continued rehabilitation on my leg, things were moving along at a steady pace as the year was coming to an end. While rehabilitating that winter, I was doing seated leg presses when I heard a soft pop with a slight jerk in my hip. I instantly knew something had happen, but I did not know what. I decided to go back to the trauma doctor to see what was going on and learned that I broke a screw at the top of the rod. The option the doctor gave me was that we could remove the screw and allow the bone to compress to see if that would help the healing. I agreed to the surgery. After having the surgery and being placed in a room, the resident rehabilitation personnel came to my room and told me I would have to stand up and try to walk as soon as possible. When I stood up, with the aid of the therapist, and started to put pressure on my leg, I instantly felt my body shift down and pain went to my hip. The pain came from the rod shifting out of the top of my femur to where the joint of my hip was. When I stood up, the screw was holding the top half of the femur in place so that the rod would not go anywhere. Without that screw in place, the rod was able to move up while the top half of the femur was stationary which meant my leg became slightly shorter than the other. The femur halves were now touching, and the hopes of my break being healed would have to start over as the year closed out.

The following year, I was still trying to find my confidence in being a breast cancer survivor. I remained focus on trying to live life as normal as possible. That also meant that I would continue to pursue happiness by finding that right woman. Things did not work out with the lady I was seeing during my cancer battle. She decided to back away from me for whatever reasons she had. Although devastated, I could not allow the emotional and physical hurt to define my future. I would continue to maintain my tenacity to move forward. I decided to pursue another young, phenomenal woman whom I had known since college. This was another time that I had to overcome my reluctance and fear to start something new. My previous relationship allowed me to be comfortable with the person who was there while I was going through the cancer. Now I had to be willing to open up for the first time and try to build something new with someone who had no idea of my cancer battle and my rehabilitation from the accident.

From the time that I had the screw removed to the time that I had to have another surgery to replace the hardware with another rod and added plate, I was in pain for approximately two years. My leg still had the break and did not seem to be healing properly. I was literally walking around on a broken leg, and it was very painful. It was tough to deal with the pain for every hour I was awake—and many of my sleepless hours. I did not let this deter me from my goals of pursuing a relationship.

I remember I would go on dates with my old friend, and it was hard enough to walk up to the restaurant from the parking lot. For her birthday, I had decided to take her to a show out of town that was on a Friday. We met up after work, and I drove us one and a half hours to the neighboring state to have a nice dinner before the show. We then went to the show, and I drove back late that night. I could not take any pain pills that entire time as I had to make sure not to get sleepy. We had a great time while we were there, but I learned how far I could really push myself. Although we had great times when we were together, we mutually decided that it was not our time, and we would remain friends. The times we spent together were great for my morale, but it manifested my physical endurance capacity.

I always tested my physical endurance during my recovery periods. I continually tested my maximum to see the progress I was making from not having to take chemical therapy treatments any longer. I remained vigilant in having the engineering camp, which accrued an awful lot of walking and standing on a broken leg. I would work on my vehicles and my house as much as I could. It was very hard to get underneath cars. It was extremely hard to get in the attic and run wires for the light fixtures I was replacing in the house and adding to the external parts of the house. You should try navigating inside the ceiling when you have a broken leg, and you have to use mostly upper body strength to get around. I cannot say that you really get used to the pain, you just deal with it and keep going. This is the mentality that was exacerbated during my cancer battle. You find ways to cope with the issues that you encounter.

I tried to find anything soothing to help deal with the constant pain coming from my leg. During the year that I had the screw removed that caused so much pain, and the following year included, I slept on an air mattress in my man cave because it did not have as much pressure on my leg as my bed's mattress. It was difficult most days having to get up and down from the floor, but at least I could sleep better at night.

After having to deal with the pain for a little over a year and no luck with the femur bone healing, my trauma doctor gave me the option of exchanging the hardware. So at the top of the next calendar year, I had the rod exchanged with a larger rod and a plate installed across the femur break. I remember waking up from that surgery and not feeling any pain in my leg when I moved it from side to side. I was looking up at my mother and my new lady friend when I started tearing up because I was not in pain anymore. Just to finally have relief from having constant and, oftentimes, excruciating pain was as close to being in heaven that I had ever been. This would be my last surgery, and I finally would be allowed to get back to the gym.

After about four months of rehabilitation for my last surgery, I was able to get back in the gym. I remember it like it was yesterday. I was so nervous to have to go and take a shower and all the guys would see my scars. My chest looked different now. I woke up early that morning with my gym bag ready to go. I went to the gym and got my gloves out. I put my work clothes and bag in the locker and had a decent workout.

When it was time to go take a shower, it felt like I had to walk a green mile. I remember getting my stuff out the locker and sitting on the bench with my head down. I was tired true enough, but my head was hanging so I could get my confidence up. "You have to do it," I whispered to myself, so I got up, pulled my shirt off, and then undressed down to my boxers. I got out my towel and soap and headed to the showers. As I came back to my locker with my towel wrapped around my waist, soap in one hand and my face towel in the other, I noticed some guys cutting eyes at my chest. As everyone was getting dressed, one of the elder men cordially asked me was I in the military. I told him no. He asked how I got the scars. I told him I was a breast cancer survivor. When the words came out of my mouth, I saw in my peripheral a few of the guys turn around. The guy I was talking to said that he recognized those scars because he only knew of one other man in his life that had breast cancer. He then asked me how I found it. I briefly told him my story while some of the other guys started listening. It was amazing how the guys started congratulating me on my survival and courage. I instantaneously started feeling good that I was not publicly ridiculed. I am sure there were more questions that they wanted to ask but just did not. Although it's true that people of all ages can be cruel, I have yet to encounter anyone who has said anything negative to me about my breast cancer survival. There are still a lot of good people out there who will continually encourage you.

Lifting weights was just the beginning of my road to recovery. My next step was trying to run to play basketball again. When I returned to the court, it truly felt like I had to learn how to run again as if I was kid learning how to walk. It was very difficult. I could barely get my legs to move as my mind was telling them to. I could barely get up and down the court. I had little side to side mobility. It took some time, but I finally got back close to about 90% after about two and half years. Things have been progressively getting better. I have been getting my life back to where it was so I can embark on my new endeavors.

CHAPTER 8 | DIVINE APPOINTMENT

The late Stuart Scott of ESPN had a seven-year battle with cancer. Scott stated that every person in the world has to "Own Your Moments." This is the perfect description of how I took control of my life-changing situation. I often call my situation my Divine Appointment. I may have asked God in the beginning "Why me?" My immediate response at the time was "Why not me?" I had to accept my calling because I had a greater calling. My family does not have a history of breast cancer. I don't carry the gene for breast cancer. I was a minority male in his early thirties that found out that he had breast cancer. According to the American Cancer Society, 2,350 new cases of invasive breast cancer are diagnosed annually. About 440 men will die from breast cancer. Breast cancer is about 100 times less common among men than women. Although these numbers do not seem like a lot, when you look at hundreds of millions in the population, there are still reasons to speak out regarding awareness.

My new life is that of a public speaker that brings awareness to breast cancer and being a motivational speaker to cancer warriors. It all started after I finished my chemical therapy treatment and was at church in October 2010, which is breast cancer awareness month. There was a breast cancer awareness presentation during the service, and they asked all the breast cancer survivors to stand. At first, I did not stand, but as I talked myself into being courageous and being a vessel for God to use, I stood up. At that moment, my life would take yet another path. I attended the CanSurvive Support Group meeting. While there, I was asked to share my story, and I did. One of the members was so intrigued with my story she told me about an upcoming event at another church and said she would share my information. She then made the statement, "I hope you are ready to go to work."

My public speaking about breast cancer has come as a whirlwind. After standing up in church, then attending a meeting, I was invited to speak at another church in the city. While I was presenting, there was a lady in the audience who was so moved by my presentation that she asked me to speak at her Foundation's Banquet that was created in honor of her daughter whom she lost to breast cancer just a few years earlier. The Kimberly Fails Jones Foundation has been such an awesome organization that gives back to the people who are suffering and struggling through cancer treatments and recovery. I agreed to be the keynote speaker for the banquet. During the time before the banquet, I was asked to do an interview with our local paper. I met the reporter at Arby's, and we sat to have a conversation regarding my breast cancer experience. After the hourlong conversation, she asked me to send her some specific pictures, so I did. I was thinking that it would eventually be a little excerpt in the paper somewhere when it was printed.

While sitting in church the following Sunday, one of the members got up with a paper in her hand to make an additional announcement.

"For those of you that did not know," she began, "there is a story about one of our members on the front page of today's paper."

When she said my name, my mouth dropped. I immediately looked at my mother who was sitting next to me. She asked me when I did the interview. I told her just the other day, but I had no clue that it was going to be on the front page. After service, I went to get a paper so I could see the article and purchased about five papers. My smile nearly broke my jaw after reading the article. I then looked at my email to find the reporter's contact information and found the email that said that the article would be featured in the state's website. It turned out that every major newspaper in the state had my article on the front page. By that afternoon, I started getting text messages and phone calls from people all over the state who saw my picture in their local paper. This was a prelude to all of my great experiences speaking out about breast cancer awareness.

I have been invited to speak at different venues all over the country to bring awareness to the growing disease. All these venues that I speak at have brought another valued memory. Each event may have its own theme that I have customized my presentation for, but the overall message is the same. You have to evaluate your strengths within and capitalize upon those strengths. You have to transform your way of thinking to handle the emotional, physical, and spiritual battle that you will encounter. As part of your preparation, it is critical to remove as much negative energy as possible. This may mean that you need to increase separation between yourself and those who are closer to you. Replace that negative energy with positive energy.

Remember that there will be people whom you will not have to remove because they will remove themselves. Some of those individuals you may want around you in a greater capacity, but they will fail to do so. These people are pieces of the puzzle that have their own place in your life, but those places are just not exactly where you would like for them to reside. Don't be discouraged or mad because they are not where you desired them to be in your life. People are wired how they are wired because of their experiences before that moment.

Chemical therapy is physically hard on the body. Try to get your body in the best fighting shape as it can be by dieting and exercise. There will unique side effects from chemical therapy for each person that will not directly resemble those of the next patient. However, there are some side effects that are consistent for most patients. Feeling sick, losing hair all over your body, and having random aches/pains are normal because of the chemicals often used for battling breast cancer. If you ever have to take the Red Devil chemical, be prepared to possibly losing your hair and having red urine immediately following consumption. Your skin hue may change, and your knuckles may become dark around the joints. Beware of getting "Chemo Brain" and becoming aggressive to people in your immediate space. Chemical therapy and radiation are not always necessary. For example, I did not need radiation, but I chose to do chemical therapy. If you have to have chemical therapy, I do recommend getting a port put in your chest so that you don't need so many needle insertions into your arms. The port makes things so much easier. The port will only leave about a one-inch scar where the incision was placed for the port.

The double mastectomy left two scars on my chest. I did not have reconstruction surgery on my chest. But I know for women, it is a much-concentrated decision to make. There is so much weight put on how people look, especially women. Beauty is only skin deep. The real beauty of a person can be found within. Look at the strength of these women and men who have to fight this fight. The emotional strength that they must have to endure the emotional and physical rollercoaster that occurs while taking chemical therapy. There will be a lot of bad days. The number of good days is dependent upon you making the most of each day.

Every day is a good day. No longer do I take the small things for granted. I loved being outside before having to fight breast cancer, but now the colors of the world are even more beautiful than before. Every breath is to be cherished, and I value the relationships for what they are when they are. There is a saying that people are in your life for a season, a reason, or a lifetime. There is even a simpler way to look at it. People in your life are either a lesson or a blessing. Evaluate, remember, and move forward. Never forget who you are and be strong. Look back into upbringing and immerse yourself into the life lessons you learned along the way and those that will have a new meaning to life as you travel the road of cancer survival. I truly try to bring a smile to everyone I encounter. We never know what a person is going through, so if I can bring a moment of joy by giving a compliment or being my normal overly charming self, then that is what I will do.

Joy is hard to come by when you are going through any cancer experience. So many questions and negative thoughts will enter your mind. You cannot go through it alone. I used to think that being alone will make you strong. In some instances, that is true, but it is so much easier when you have a support cast. Love and affection go a long way to enforce the positive energy that surrounds you. That is why it so good to see smiling faces from people who work at the hospitals and clinics like Clearview Cancer Institute. Cancer warriors value those moments to see a smiling face or converse with people who genuinely care. Even hobbies will bring you joy.

I have been fortunate that my hobbies have brought me new friends and colleagues. Being able to get back in the gym, play basketball, and ride my motorcycle has established new friendships and reconnected old ones. My speaking engagements have brought new friendships as well as an increased pink tie and accessories wardrobe. I get a lot of satisfaction out of being debonair. However, I get the most satisfaction getting back to playing sports. I get to meet so many people and try to bring awareness wherever I go. One of my most memorable moments in getting back to playing basketball was one October; the guys surprised me with everyone wearing pink one particular day. They secretly orchestrated the pink representation that Saturday in honor of me. We even took pictures that day. I know a majority of those guys from playing ball only. I have a lot of respect for what they did. Moments like that are what make me keep speaking out about breast cancer awareness. I remember one lady kept a cut out of my article in her purse for over a year until I was able to come and speak at a local event. She said I was so much of an inspiration to her. I recall another moment when I had just delivered a speech in another town, and as I was taking questions, a lady expressed her admiration for what I was doing. As she explained her cancer experience, she was telling me about how much she admired my courage to stand up and talk about my cancer victory. It is so hard for people to talk about it, and they sit in silence so long not talking about this disease that could be killing them. This is why you have to talk and open up. Tell people about what you are going through. Stress can also damage the body. Silence is an added threat to the battle against cancer. You don't have to go through it alone. There are so many people that you may or may not know who depend on you being around. I have learned that there are people always watching when you don't believe they are watching. There are people who are willing to do whatever they can to help you make it through. They may not know what to say, but if you just signal out to them for help, they will be there. I remember telling one of my professional colleagues in NSBE that I needed some personal items. He and his wife quickly brought them over. I had almost all of my NSBE family come and visit me at one time or another.

The main thing about fighting any type of cancer (a disease or a situation) is that you have to take control of the battle. You have to understand that you have a destiny and a purpose. To fulfill your purpose efficiently, you have to go through your battle to the best of your ability. You have to reshape your mentality and take hold of the situation and attack it head-on. Be positive in your display and believe that you have victory. Your victory will benefit so many people—and some of them will be people you didn't even know were cheering for you. Oftentimes, in a sparring match between two gladiators, the winner is announced after the fight. You are divinely appointed as the winner before the fight occurs, in whatever capacity that is. You are getting ready to go through the battle, but this battle goes beyond your moments, and you have already won the battle. Don't wait until the end of the race to raise your hand as the winner of this contest. Smile and raise your hand now. You have already won because you chose to fight. Congratulations, the champion is you–the warrior who is directly changing the world through your influence on the people who watch and cheer for you.

ABOUT THE AUTHOR

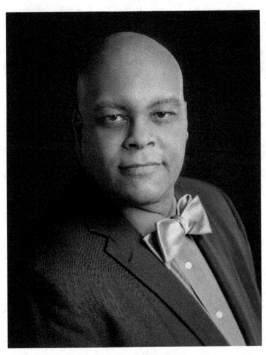

Derrick Cameron was born in Mount Holly, New Jersey. He has lived in different cultures around the world. He is the product of a single parent home, but he has always been active in sports. He is a dual graduate of the University of Alabama in Huntsville (UAH). Derrick has served the Huntsville community in several capacities. He has served on the executive board for the National Society of Black Engineers (NSBE) for both the UAH chapter and the North Alabama Professionals chapter. Derrick initiated a free weeklong Summer Engineering Camp for 500 kids with the assistance of Dr. Terrance West and Latoya Eggleston. He has also served on the Science, Technology, Engineering, and Math (STEM) Outreach Boards for Sierra Lobo and the National Defense Industrial Association–Tennessee Valley Chapter. He still enjoys playing sports, riding motorcycles, and participating in outdoor recreations.

CPSIA information can be obtained
at www.ICGtesting.com
Printed in the USA
LVHW021507141120
671494LV00006B/777

9 781735 645902